THE FRACTURED SCAPHOID

THE FRACTURED SCAPHOID

TIMOTHY J. HERBERT
M.B., B.S., F.R.C.S., F.R.A.C.S.

Orthopaedic Surgeon,
Sydney Hospital Hand Unit,
Sydney, New South Wales,
Australia

with 255 *illustrations*

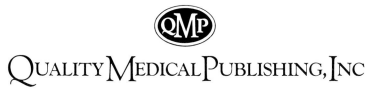

QUALITY MEDICAL PUBLISHING, INC

ST. LOUIS, MISSOURI
1990

PUBLISHER'S NOTE At the author's request, British spellings have been used throughout this book. The terms "doctor" and "surgeon," rather than "physician," have been used in keeping with British usage.

Copyright © 1990 by Quality Medical Publishing, Inc.

All rights reserved. Reproduction of the material herein in any form requires the written permission of the publisher.

Printed in the United States of America.

PUBLISHER Karen Berger
ASSOCIATE EDITOR Beth Campbell
PROJECT MANAGER Carlotta Seely
PRODUCTION Susan Trail, Judy Bamert
COVER DESIGN Diane M. Beasley
BOOK DESIGN Susan Trail
ILLUSTRATOR Vicki M. Friedman

Quality Medical Publishing, Inc.
2086 Craigshire Drive
St. Louis, Missouri 63146

LIBRARY OF CONGRESS CATALOGING IN PUBLICATION DATA

Herbert, Timothy J., 1941-
  The fractured scaphoid / Timothy J. Herbert.
    p.   cm.
  Includes bibliographical references.
  Includes index.
  ISBN 0-942219-06-6 (hardcover)
  1. Scaphoid bone—Fractures—Treatment. 2. Internal fixation in fractures. I. Title.
  [DNLM: 1. Carpal Bones—surgery. 2. Fractures—surgery. 3. Wrist Injuries. WE 830 H537f]
RD559.H47   1990
617.1'57—dc20
DNLM/DLC
for Library of Congress   90-8800
                                                              CIP

VT/WW/WW
5   4   3   2   1

Foreword

This book is different from most that you have read. Critics will say that it is unscientific, anecdotal, and sparsely referenced. All of that may be true, but it is also a very important book, for it contains the philosophy and concepts developed from the vast clinical experience of an orthopaedic surgeon with solid credentials. Tim Herbert has undoubtedly operated on more patients with scaphoid nonunion than anyone in the world, and that alone makes it imperative that he share his experience with us. More important, however, he has studied, pondered, and thought exhaustively about the scaphoid for nearly 20 years. He is a very bright, impeccably honest, and highly innovative surgeon who has effectively used his enormous clinical experience as an ongoing search for better ways of treating difficult wrist problems. This book is *not* about a gimmick, and it is *not* intended as a marketing ploy to sell more Herbert screws. Rather, it is an extremely thoughtful dissertation that should be read, reread, and contemplated by all surgeons who deal with this tiny carpal bone that has fascinated and challenged orthopaedic and hand surgeons for decades.

One of the delightful features of this book is that it is easy and fun to read. The manuscript arrived on my desk at a particularly busy time for me, and I intended to merely skim the text before writing this foreword. Even though I have heard Dr. Herbert speak about the scaphoid on several occasions and I have had many conversations with him about the subject, I immediately found myself engrossed in his highly readable, very personal style, and I thoroughly enjoyed every word of the manuscript. It is replete with pearls about the concepts of scaphoid fractures, the decision-making process associated with these fractures, and the technical details of operative treatment.

Foreword

As the author himself acknowledges, many of the problems of the scaphoid remain unsolved, but in sharing his thoughts with us he has lifted our understanding of the scaphoid to a higher level. Others will take his ideas, modify and build upon them, and we shall continue to improve our knowledge of this intriguing little bone, with thanks to Tim Herbert for his valuable contributions to that quest.

David P. Green, M.D.

Preface

When I was first approached about writing a book on scaphoid fractures, my initial reaction was a negative one for two reasons. The first was purely personal. I prefer sailing to writing! The second reason was more formidable: I questioned the need for such a book. So much has been written already about this fracture, and recent publications on wrist surgery appear to cover the subject more than adequately. What, then, led me to change my mind? I believe it was the conviction that we need to rethink our whole approach to the management of this common injury and to try and shake off some of those outdated concepts that still influence much of our current thinking on this subject.

Every senior medical student is aware of the problems associated with a missed diagnosis, and all orthopaedic surgeons have been firmly indoctrinated in the necessity for early and prolonged immobilisation when treating scaphoid fractures. The following anecdote illustrates the extent of this indoctrination. A surgical examinee was being questioned on the management of scaphoid fractures. Quite correctly he prescribed a scaphoid cast with review after 6 weeks. "And if the fracture has not healed?" asked the examiner. "Then I would reapply the plaster for another 6 weeks," came the reply. "And what if the fracture remains ununited?" "Then I would reapply the plaster for another 6 weeks." The same question and answer were repeated several more times before the examiner, in desperation, asked the student how much longer he intended to continue this treatment in the absence of any radiological evidence of union. "Until the bell rings" was the reply!

Whether or not this story is true, it emphasises the focus of conventional teaching on the importance of repetitive and prolonged immobilisation of the wrist in the treatment of this injury. More than 30 years ago, McLaughlin* challenged this approach, but little heed of his message was taken, and current practise accepts that at least 90% of scaphoid fractures do heal uneventfully with conservative treatment.

Some 20 years ago, during my orthopaedic training in London, I became concerned about the number of patients attending outpatient clinics with nonunion of the scaphoid. A retrospective study of 200 acute scaphoid fractures, treated conservatively, suggested that the longer a fracture needed to be immobilised, the less likely it was to unite. Furthermore, there appeared to be a correlation between the incidence of nonunion and the radiological appearance of the acute fracture: several clearly recognisable fracture types (unstable fractures) were associated with an increased risk of nonunion.† Encouraged by mentors who taught me that there is always more than one way to treat any orthopaedic problem, I started to question the validity of the conventional approach to scaphoid fracture management. Further encouraged by the "Pyrford principle," which states that "joints are supposed to move," I became interested in the concept of internal fixation as an alternative method of treating the acute scaphoid fracture. I soon learned, as others have learned before me, that trying to internally fix an unstable scaphoid fracture can be a humiliating experience. This motivated me to search for a better technique for internal fixation of the scaphoid bone.

I do not wish this book to be seen as a vehicle for promoting the instrumentation that was developed following this research. Rather, I wish to share the lessons I have learned, sometimes painfully, as a result of operating on more than 500 scaphoid fractures during the last 10 years. The majority of these procedures have been for established nonunion and other complications; my experience with acute scaphoid fractures remains relatively limited. Whenever possible, I have tried to obtain the original x-ray films and accurate histories from patients. These studies have taught me much about the natural history of scaphoid fractures.

---

*McLaughlin HL. Fractures of the carpal navicular (scaphoid) bone: Some observations based on treatment by open reduction and internal fixation. J Bone Joint Surg 36A:763, 1954.
†Herbert TJ. Scaphoid fractures and carpal instability. Proc R Soc Med 67:1080, 1974.

In this book I have approached the problem of the fractured scaphoid from the viewpoint of a practising clinician who, at times, has allowed himself to be influenced by his patients. I have therefore excluded reference to much of the excellent experimental work that has been carried out in recent years and has taught us so much about the anatomy and biomechanics of the wrist. I have included only those references that have a direct bearing on treatment. I have included short chapters on unusual aspects of scaphoid injuries such as malunion, fractures in the skeletally immature, and ligamentous damage leading to rotary instability. Of necessity, my experience in these areas remains limited and most of this work is previously unpublished. However, all new techniques are the subject of carefully controlled clinical trials, and the results will be published once sufficient experience and follow-up have been achieved. Some of the ideas expressed in this book may be viewed as controversial. Not everyone will agree with them; indeed, I would be disappointed if this were the case. However, an open mind is a fertile mind, and perhaps a few of the seeds sown in this small book will reach fruition.

It is a singular honour that Dr. David Green has written the foreword to this volume. Dr. Green is not only a world authority on the scaphoid but also is a master in the art of medical writing. Thus, whilst making me aware of this book's many deficiencies, he nonetheless encouraged me to publish it by sharing with me his philosophy: "A book is never completed—it is simply abandoned!"

As I "abandon" this text, I would like to thank Karen Berger and the rest of the QMP staff for their help, support, and gentle persuasiveness. My secretaries, Chris Sturt and Phoebe Cleary, have accepted with good humour the prolonged absences from my true place of duty that often arise when one is involved in clinical research and teaching. This book could never have been written without their invaluable help, since they are, perhaps, the only people in the world who can decipher my handwriting! My wife, Heidi, has continued to teach me how to keep things in true perspective and has been a constant support. I am indebted to my medical colleagues in Australia who have consistently referred patients to me for treatment. Finally, I wish to thank the patients themselves, who have taught me so much and to whom this book is dedicated.

Timothy J. Herbert

Contents

1. A Single Small Bone, 1

2. Anatomy and Biomechanics, 11
   - Osteology, 12
   - Ligamentous Attachments, 14
   - Blood Supply, 14
   - Functional Anatomy, 16
   - Mechanism of Injury, 20

3. Diagnosis, 27
   - History of Injury, 28
   - Examination, 30
   - Radiographical Examination, 32
   - Other Imaging Techniques, 38

4. Natural History, 43

5. A Rational Approach to Treatment of Acute Scaphoid Fractures, 51
   - Stable Fractures, 52
   - "Clinical" Fractures, 56
   - Tubercle Fractures, 57
   - Unstable Fractures, 57
   - Classification of Scaphoid Fractures, 62

6. Acute Fractures and Delayed Union: Surgical Techniques, 69
   - Surgical Approaches to the Scaphoid, 70
   - Fracture Reduction, 76
   - Internal Fixation, 77
   - Postoperative Management, 84
   - Results and Complications, 88

7. Treatment of Established Nonunion, 91
   - Staging of Scaphoid Nonunions, 94
   - Treatment of Fibrous Union, 96
   - Treatment of Scaphoid Pseudarthrosis, 100
   - Scaphoid Reconstruction, 103
   - Small Proximal Pole Fractures, 112

8. Avascular Necrosis of the Scaphoid, 121
   - Diagnosis, 124
   - Treatment, 126
   - Partial Silastic Replacement, 131
   - Results and Complications, 136

9 Salvage Procedures for
  Scaphoid Nonunion, 139

  Radial Styloidectomy, 140
  Osteophyte Excision, 143
  Wrist Denervation, 145
  Scaphoid Arthroplasty and Limited
    Intercarpal Fusion, 145
  Proximal Row Carpectomy, 150
  Wrist Fusion, 151

10 Scaphoid Malunion, 155

  Diagnosis, 157
  Management, 159
  Surgical Technique, 159
  Results and Complications, 161

11 Scaphoid Fractures in the
  Skeletally Immature, 163

  Diagnosis, 166
  Management, 166
  Complications, 170

12 Rotary Subluxation of the
  Scaphoid, 173

  Diagnosis, 180
  Management, 184
  Surgical Technique, 184

  The Future, 193

  Index, 195

THE FRACTURED SCAPHOID

1

A Single Small Bone

. . . To teach that over 90% of acute scaphoid fractures will heal without complication after conservative treatment is misleading, if not dangerous.

Chapter 1

At last count the adult skeleton contained at least 206 separate bones. One of the smallest of these is the carpal scaphoid. (I prefer the Greek term "scaphoid" to the Latin term "navicular" for the simple reason that it has two fewer syllables.) Why devote an entire book to fractures of this single, small, and seemingly insignificant bone? The fact is that the problems and morbidity associated with fractures of the scaphoid bear no relationship to its size. For the patient whose limb is immobilised in a plaster cast for 3 or 4 months, the size, shape, or name of the fractured bone matters little.

For a moment let us consider the fractured scaphoid from the patient's point of view. Imagine the following scenario: a healthy young man falls heavily onto his outstretched hand whilst playing football on Saturday afternoon.* He immediately dismisses the acute pain as a "sprain." He does not hear a crack, the limb does not become unstable, and he is able to complete the game. By evening his wrist is swollen and motion is somewhat restricted. However, with the use of ice, analgesics, and an elastic bandage, the pain settles and he returns to work on Monday morning.

One of several things may then happen. The man's wrist may continue to improve with time and he forgets the injury. Months or even years later he becomes aware of pain and weakness in the wrist, possibly as a result of further trauma. X-ray films are taken and show evidence of an old ununited fracture of the scaphoid (Figure 1-1). If his symptoms are severe enough, he will be faced with reconstructive surgery and several months away from work. If he is more fortunate, he may never know that he has had a fractured scaphoid, although he may complain of a little "arthritis" in his wrist as the years go by, which he uses as a convenient excuse for his increasing golf handicap.

Alternatively, persistent pain and swelling may prompt the patient to seek medical attention shortly after the injury. Once acute tenderness in the anatomical snuff-box has been demonstrated, radiographs are requested. Here chance plays a major role. It is possible that the x-ray film may not show a fracture, in which case the patient may be

---

*Men are used in patient profiles throughout the book because they represent the overwhelming majority of cases of scaphoid fractures.

sent home without further treatment. However, if he consults a vigilant doctor, he will be told that a plaster should be applied as a precautionary measure. Although the patient complies readily, he may wonder why he needs a plaster cast when the bone is not actually broken. Once he finds just how difficult life can be with the wrist and thumb immobilised in plaster, he may start to question the wisdom of the treatment, particularly when he has to stay home from work, with no money coming in to pay the mortgage. At this stage the strong-willed or desperate individual may take matters into his own hands, remove the plaster, and quietly forget about the next appointment with the doctor. A more compliant patient will tolerate the inconvenience of the cast until he is told that the

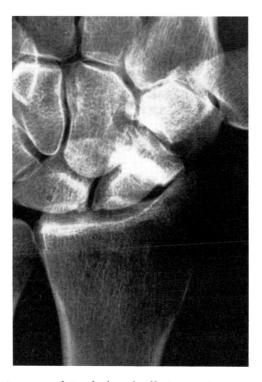

Figure 1-1. This patient complained of gradually increasing pain and stiffness in the left wrist but was unable to recall a specific injury. X-ray studies show an established scaphoid nonunion; osteoarthritic changes indicate that this fracture has been present for some years.

Chapter 1

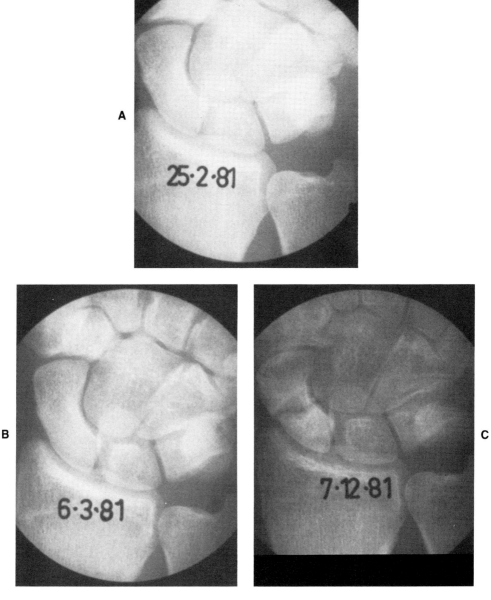

Figure 1-2. **A,** Initial radiograph at the time of injury showed no evidence of fracture. **B,** Repeat x-rays taken 2 weeks later again fail to show a fracture. **C,** Radiograph taken 9 months later; established nonunion is now apparent.

A Single Small Bone

x-ray result is clear and he is discharged from treatment. Of course, this does not mean that the scaphoid has not been fractured; an established nonunion may become apparent months or even years later (Figure 1-2).

A third possibility is that a fracture of the scaphoid may be confirmed at the second x-ray examination. The patient is told that the cast must stay on for at least another 6 weeks. Provided he has faith in his doctor and that his financial and sporting demands are not overwhelming, he will comply with this treatment in the absolute belief that *all fractures heal when immobilised in a plaster cast*. What is he to believe when further review suggests that all is not well? If the doctor recommends continued immobilisation, the patient starts to question how this treatment can be effective when it failed to heal the fracture before. Alternatively, if surgery is suggested, the patient wonders why this treatment was not recommended in the first place, thus saving him the inconvenience of 8 or more weeks of fruitless treatment (Figure 1-3). If, as so often happens, the treating doctor appears to be somewhat uncertain, who can blame the patient for terminating treatment?

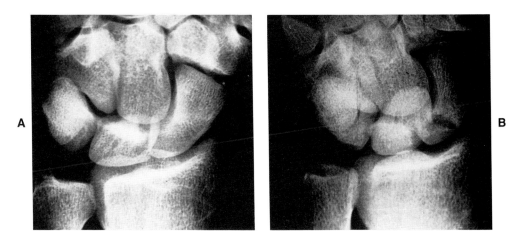

Figure 1-3. A, This patient sought treatment in April 1988 for an acute injury to his dominant left wrist. X-ray examination showed an undisplaced fracture through the proximal pole of the scaphoid. **B,** X-ray appearance after 3 months of continuous immobilisation in a plaster cast. The x-ray film shows clear signs of nonunion for which surgery is indicated.

Chapter 1

Finally, there is the patient in whom the fracture has been diagnosed from the outset and who has sufficient faith in his doctor to comply with whatever treatment is imposed. He understands that he will need to spend at least 8 to 12 weeks in a plaster cast, although it may prevent him from working. Even if the patient is aware of the muscle wasting and joint stiffness that may occur during immobilisation, he complies, believing firmly that the outcome will be a normal wrist. What if after 3 months he is told that the cast must be reapplied or, worse still, that he needs an operation followed by 3 more months in a plaster cast? Having already invested so much time in this form of treatment, how can the patient now refuse? Let us hope, in this case, that the outcome of surgery is successful.

These scenarios are not imaginary; they are based on numerous case histories and discussions with patients referred to me for treatment of complications after conservative treatment of scaphoid fractures. It is not hard to sympathise with those patients who wish that they had never had their wrist radiographed in the first place!

Many acute scaphoid fractures heal uneventfully with conservative treatment. Some develop a fibrous union, whereas others, perhaps the majority, develop an unstable nonunion and increasing deformity of the scaphoid, ultimately leading to osteoarthritis of the wrist.

Although scaphoid fracture following a fall on the outstretched hand is undoubtedly the most common fracture in young adults, the true incidence of this injury remains unknown, since so many patients pass the original injury off as a simple sprain. A comprehensive epidemiological study is needed to determine the true frequency of scaphoid fractures and their complications. However, if one assumes an incidence of 1 in 50 of the population at risk (I know of no football team that does not have at least one player with a scaphoid fracture) and that the average time lost from work for treatment is 12 weeks, then in a country the size of Australia fractures of this single small bone alone could account for well up to 500,000 man-hours lost per year. In a survey on the frequency and cost of upper extremity disorders in the United States,[1] the incidence of carpal fractures and dislocations was estimated at more than 500,000 per year, resulting in more than 3.5 million days lost from work. This figure compares unfavourably with all other fractures, except perhaps for those involving the spine and skull, whose devastating effects are the result of associated nerve damage.

In Sydney I see about 50 new patients a year who have symptomatic nonunion of the scaphoid. These patients are drawn from a population of approximately 6 million people, and of course I see only a small percentage of the total number of patients with this problem. Of interest, however, is the fact that at least half of these patients have already received treatment for their original fracture. In many cases the treatment was supervised by an orthopaedic surgeon and consisted of plaster immobilisation until the fracture was considered healed. The average period of wrist immobilisation in a plaster cast is about 12 weeks, ranging from a few days at one extreme to more than 18 months at the other. Nearly all of these patients say that their wrist "never felt right" after treatment but accepted a degree of discomfort and weakness as a trade-off for returning to normal activities. When the original x-ray films were available, I have been impressed by how difficult it is to determine when a scaphoid fracture has healed after treatment with plaster casting. In some cases the fracture line is never distinct, and yet the patient returns a year or two later with clear radiological evidence of an established nonunion (Figure 1-4). In other cases the established radiological criteria for union appeared to be present, yet follow-up studies have shown clearly that this was not the case (Figure 1-5).

In other words, it may be extremely difficult, if not impossible, to determine from x-ray findings alone when a scaphoid fracture has healed.[2,3] I have reached the conclusion that *the only way to verify healing after completion of treatment is by prolonged clinical and radiological follow-up.* Only then will we know the true incidence of nonunion after conservative treatment of the acute fracture. I believe that to teach that over 90% of acute scaphoid fractures will heal without complication after conservative treatment is misleading, if not dangerous. The price for such complacency is high, since the natural history of the ununited scaphoid fracture is progressive carpal collapse deformity, leading to irreversible osteoarthritis of the wrist.

A better understanding and appreciation of the biomechanics of the scaphoid bone, the mechanism of injury, the natural history of treated and untreated fractures, and the late complications should result

Chapter 1

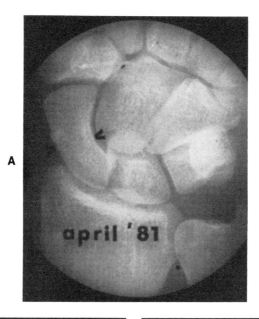
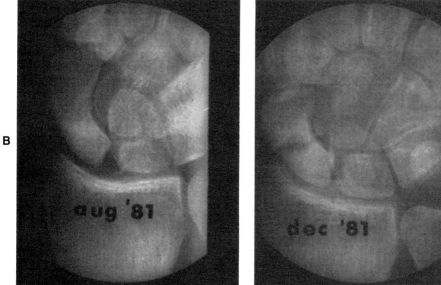

Figure 1-4. Radiographs of a patient who sought treatment for symptomatic nonunion. **A,** Original films showed a minor stable fracture. **B,** After treatment in a plaster cast for several months, the fracture appeared soundly healed. **C,** The patient presented in December 1981 with symptomatic nonunion. (From Herbert TJ, Fisher WE. Management of the fractured scaphoid using a new bone screw. J Bone Joint Surg 66B:114, 1984.)

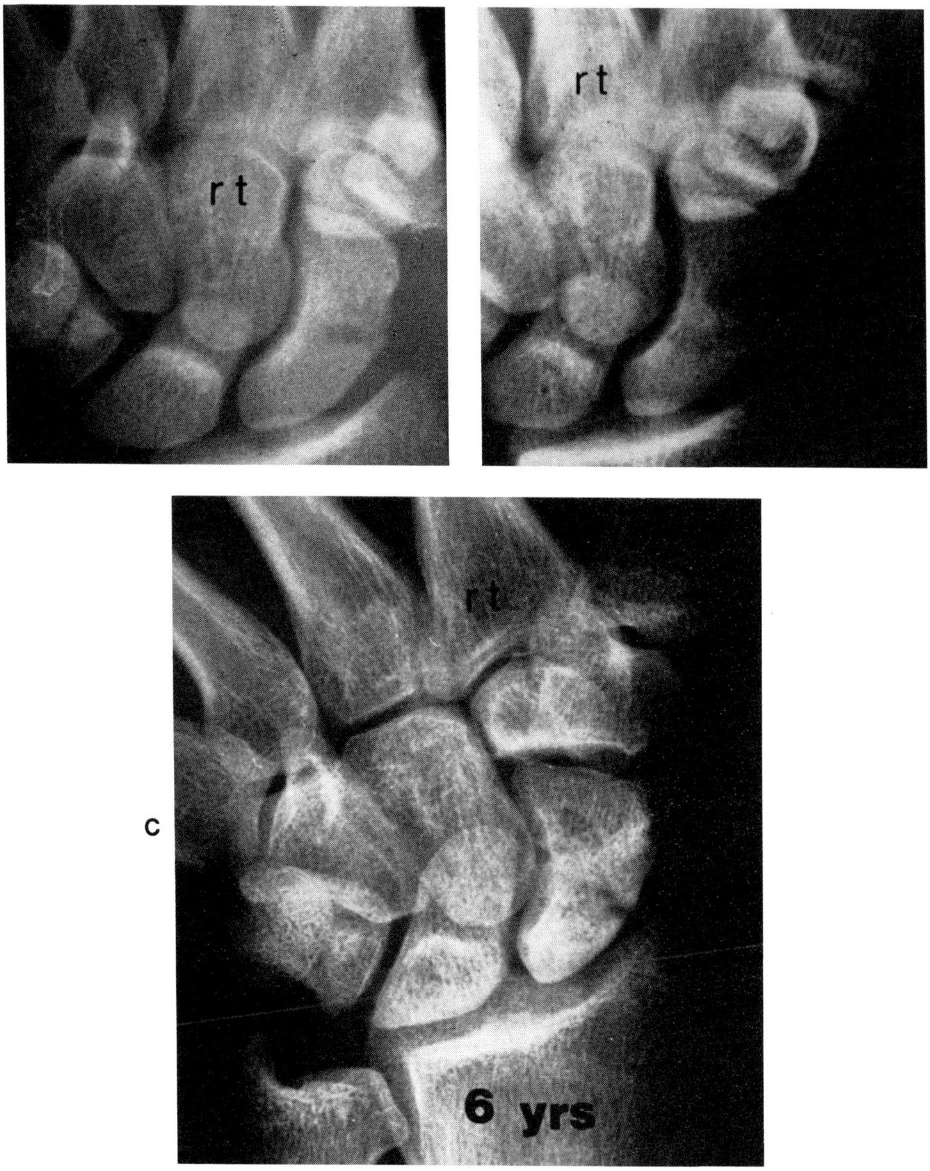

Figure 1-5. A, X-ray films of a patient with an acute fracture through the waist of the left scaphoid. **B,** X-ray appearance after cast immobilisation for 3 months. The fracture line is no longer visible and cross-trabeculation suggests that union has occurred. **C,** Six years later there is established nonunion with associated carpal collapse deformity and early osteoarthritis.

in a more rational approach to the management of this common injury.

Let us again focus on the patient. Is it not reasonable for him to demand a form of treatment that provides the best possible result, in the shortest possible time, with the least disruption in daily activity? Why should the patient accept even 1 day in plaster if this is unnecessary? On the other hand, why should he have to put up with 3 months in a plaster cast if union cannot be guaranteed at the end of that time? Should the patient have any treatment at all if his symptoms are not causing significant disability? Is there a possibility that the fracture will heal without treatment? If the patient develops a nonunion, what are the chances that this will cause significant disability? Is a nonunion after treatment any less troublesome than one occurring without treatment? If all other fractures of the wrist and hand unite in 6 weeks, why should fractures of the scaphoid be different? These questions must be examined, even if all the answers are not yet known.

In this book I have attempted to formulate a rational approach to the management of this troublesome and disabling injury based on extensive personal experience. I ask the reader to keep an open mind and, perhaps more difficult, to shed some of those old and preconceived concepts about this injury that continue to appear in much of the present literature.

REFERENCES

1. Kelsey JL, Pastides H, Kreiger N, Harris C, Chernow RA. Upper Extremity Disorders: A Survey of Their Frequency and Cost in the United States. St. Louis: CV Mosby, 1980.
2. Dias JJ, Taylor M, Thompson J, Brenkel IJ, Gregg PJ. Radiographic signs of union of scaphoid fractures: An analysis of inter-observer agreement and reproducibility. J Bone Joint Surg 70B:299, 1988.
3. Dias JJ, Brenkel IJ, Finlay DBL. Patterns of union in fractures of the waist of the scaphoid. J Bone Joint Surg 71B:307, 1989.

2

Anatomy and Biomechanics

The unique mobility of the human
wrist results from the complex articulations at
both the radiocarpal and midcarpal joints.
The price of this mobility is potential
wrist instability....

Chapter 2

OSTEOLOGY

The scaphoid is a three-dimensional bone within a three-dimensional carpus (Figure 2-1). A common error is to think of the bone in two-dimensional terms, since it appears this way on x-ray film. The result of such a misconception can be disastrous. Because neither words nor diagrams are any substitute for the real thing, I urge you to hold a model of the scaphoid bone in your hand whilst reading this chapter.

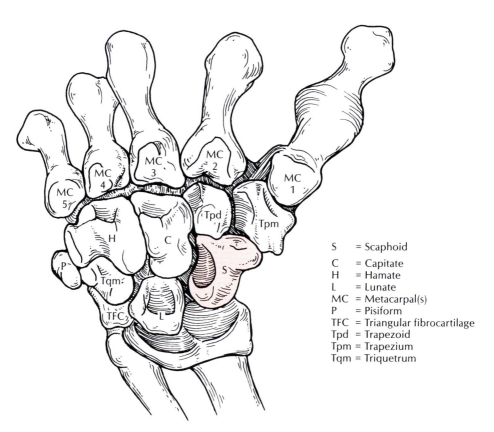

Figure 2-1. Three-dimensional relationship between the bones of the carpus. Note the inherent instability of the system. (Redrawn from Anderson JE, ed. Grant's Atlas of Anatomy, 7th ed., Baltimore: Williams & Wilkins, 1978, Fig. 6-114.)

Anatomy and Biomechanics

It is useful to think of the scaphoid as a small tubular bone that has been twisted and bent into an S shape. It lies entirely within the wrist joint, with more than 80% of its surface being covered by articular cartilage (Figure 2-2).

The scaphoid is concave on its ulnar surface, where it articulates with the capitate. Proximally it has a small, semilunar-shaped facet for articulation with the lunate. Around the borders of this facet are the scapholunate ligament attachments. The proximal third of the radial surface of the bone is convex and articulates with the radius. Distal to this articulation is the waist, grooved on its volar surface by the radioscaphocapitate ligament and ridged across the dorsoradial surface, where the capsule attaches along the edges of the spiral groove. Distal to the waist, the scaphoid expands in both directions to form the prominent tubercle on the volar surface, and the distal convex surface articulates with the trapezium and trapezoid.

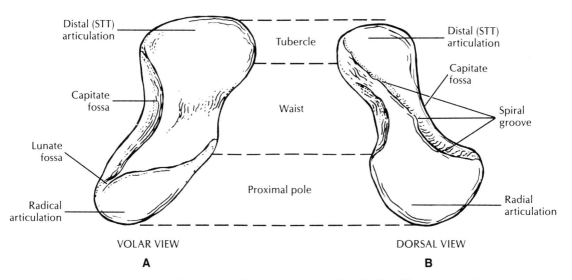

Figure 2-2. Right scaphoid. **A,** *Volar view:* Note tubercle distally, narrowed waist, and proximal pole, which articulates with the scaphoid fossa of the radius. Medially a large concave fossa articulates with the capitate. **B,** *Dorsal view:* Note the spiral groove separating the distal and proximal articular surfaces. The dorsal capsule attaches along the spiral groove and is the major source of blood supply to the scaphoid.

LIGAMENTOUS ATTACHMENTS

Although Taleisnik[1,2] and Mayfield, Johnson, and Kilcoyne[3] have in exacting detail described the complex extrinsic and intrinsic ligamentous structures of the wrist, the clinical significance of many of these structures is sometimes difficult to evaluate. I believe that the stability of the scaphoid in relation to the adjacent carpal bones depends to a great extent on the short interosseous or intrinsic ligaments that attach it distally to the trapezium and trapezoid and proximally to the lunate (Figure 2-3). Motion in both these joints is restricted by these short, strong ligaments, which allow a degree of rotation proximally and a degree of gliding distally. These ligaments merge with the extrinsic ligaments (Figure 2-4) and capsule, which are loose enough to allow free motion of the scaphoid bone within the wrist. The strong volar radioscaphocapitate ligament appears to act as a sling across the waist of the scaphoid without any obvious attachment to the bone. The radiolunate ligament acts as a "labrum" supporting the proximal pole of the scaphoid.

BLOOD SUPPLY

Elegant studies performed by Gelberman et al.[4-6] clearly demonstrate that the scaphoid receives its blood supply through the areas of soft tissue attachment. The dorsal vasculature enters through numerous small foramina along the spiral groove and dorsal ridge. These feeding vessels arise from the dorsal scaphoid branch of the radial artery and from the dorsal radial carpal arch. This source accounts for approximately 80% of the total blood supply to the scaphoid. The distal 20% of the bone is supplied by palmar vessels entering the tubercle and distal pole. Gelberman[4-6] has failed to demonstrate any intraosseous connexion between these two areas of blood supply; similarly, he has been unable to show any significant blood supply entering through the attachments of the scapholunate ligaments.

Anatomy and Biomechanics

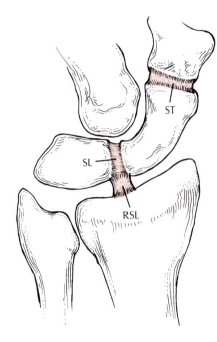

Figure 2-3. The *important* intrinsic ligaments of the scaphoid.

RSL = Radioscapholunate ligament
SL = Scapholunate ligament
ST = Scaphotrapezial ligament

RL = Radiolunate ligament
RSC = Radioscaphocapitate ligament
TCL = Transverse carpal ligament

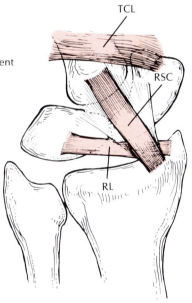

Figure 2-4. The important volar *extrinsic* ligaments of the scaphoid. Acting as a "labrum" on the volar surface of the radius, the *radiolunate* ligament supports the proximal pole of the scaphoid. The *radioscaphocapitate* ligament serves as a sling beneath the scaphoid waist. Note the attachment of the flexor retinaculum (*TCL*) onto the scaphoid tubercle.

My clinical experience does not entirely substantiate these findings. I have observed numerous patients in whom a small proximal pole fragment remains viable when the scapholunate ligament can be its only possible source of blood supply. Also, I have seen patients in whom avascular necrosis of the proximal pole has occurred after avulsion injuries of the scapholunate ligament without any associated fracture (Preiser's disease). Thus it appears that the proximal pole must receive some vascular supply through the attachments of the scapholunate ligament.

At surgery, I routinely divide the volar ligament and capsule between the scaphoid and the trapezium; I have noted no evidence of devascularisation of the scaphoid resulting from this manoeuvre, which leads me to conclude that a satisfactory intramedullary blood flow must exist within the scaphoid.

Fortunately the soft tissue attachments along the dorsal ridge are extensive and are normally spared from damage even when the scaphoid has undergone complete rotary dislocation. These soft tissue attachments are not at risk when the standard volar or a limited dorsal approach to the scaphoid is used; however, it appears that the attachments could be compromised with the dorsolateral approach sometimes recommended.

In my experience complete avascular necrosis of the proximal pole of the scaphoid is rare after a fracture unless adjacent soft tissues have sustained significant trauma either as a result of injury or surgery.

FUNCTIONAL ANATOMY

The unique mobility of the human wrist results from the complex articulations at both the radiocarpal and midcarpal joints. The price of this mobility is potential wrist instability and a tendency for the carpus to collapse under loading. The scaphoid acts as a bridge or link across the midcarpal joint (Figure 2-5). Thus any shear strain that occurs across the midcarpal joint is transferred to the scaphoid, causing it either to fracture or dislocate. Fisk[7] has clearly shown that the carpus tends to collapse if it is not supported by the scaphoid bone (Figure 2-6, A-C). When severed of its ligamentous attachments, the scaphoid assumes an anteverted position, the lunate and triquetrum subluxate forward and rotate dorsally, and the capitate and hamate subluxate dorsally and proximally, producing the so-called "dorsiflexed intercalated segment instability" (DISI) deformity. This deformity limits extension of the wrist and leads to the development of osteoarthritis as a result of abnormal loading on the articular surfaces of the midcarpal joint. It does not take long for the capsule and ligaments to contract, producing a fixed deformity as opposed to an instability (Figure 2-6, *D*).

Should an unstable fracture occur through the body of the scaphoid, the same deformity will develop (Figure 2-6, *E*). The proximal pole of the scaphoid remains attached to and moves with the lunate and triquetrum, whereas the distal pole assumes an anteverted or flexed position. If the scaphoid fracture remains unstable, the deformity increases as the carpus collapses, and wear on the impinging volar frag-

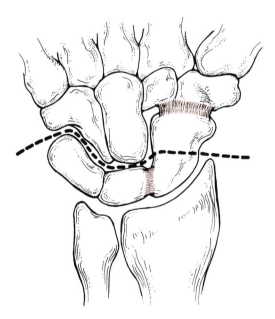

Figure 2-5. The scaphoid bone "bridges" the midcarpal joint. Because of its strong proximal and distal ligamentous attachments, the bone acts as a restraining link, preventing dislocation of the midcarpal joint. The dotted line shows how the stress axis of the midcarpal joint passes across the scaphoid waist.

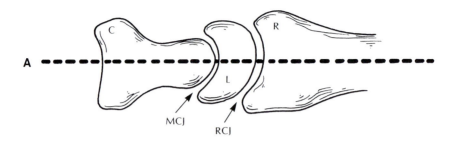

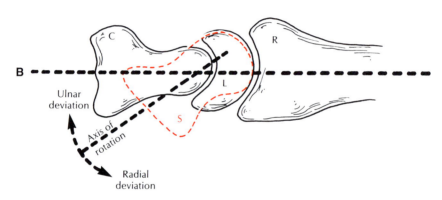

Figure 2-6. A, Lateral view of the wrist demonstrating normal carpal alignment. *C,* Capitate; *L,* lunate; *R,* radius; *RCJ,* radiocarpal joint; *MCJ,* midcarpal joint. **B,** The scaphoid bone (*S*), by means of its proximal and distal attachments, acts as a link to support the midcarpal joint. The scaphoid (and to a lesser extent the attached lunate) flexes with radial deviation and extends with ulnar deviation of the wrist. **C,** Without the scaphoid, the unsupported carpus tends to collapse into the DISI, or zig-zag, deformity. Subluxation of the midcarpal joints blocks extension of the wrist and leads to the development of osteoarthritis. **D,** When severed of its ligamentous attachments, the scaphoid assumes a flexed, or anteverted, position, allowing the carpus to collapse. **E,** An unstable scaphoid fracture results in a similar carpal collapse pattern, leading to progressive humpback deformity of the scaphoid. (Modified from Fisk GR. Carpal instability and the fractured scaphoid. Ann Roy Coll Surg Engl 46:63, 1970.)

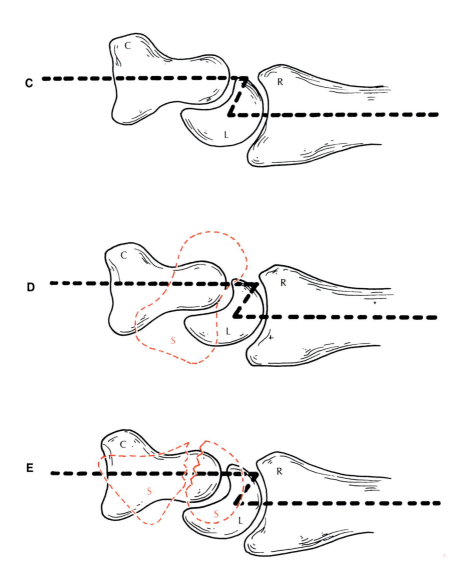

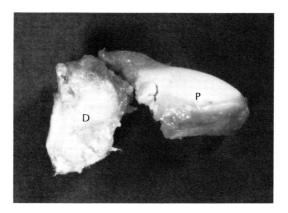

Figure 2-7. This photograph of the left carpal scaphoid bone (dorsoradial view) shows the "humpback" deformity associated with an unstable pseudarthrosis. D, Distal pole; P, proximal pole. Note displacement of the fragments with bone resorption, leading to a volar angulatory deformity and dorsal osteophyte formation.

ments of the scaphoid leads to bone resorption and further deformity (Figure 2-7). Secondary soft tissue contracture produces a fixed deformity of the carpus, causing increasing stiffness of the wrist. For this reason I prefer to use the term "carpal collapse deformity" rather than "dorsiflexed intercalated segment instability" because the latter incorrectly implies looseness or instability of the wrist.

MECHANISM OF INJURY

One only needs to hold a dry scaphoid bone in one's hand to appreciate the amount of force required to break it. In the vast majority of patients a clear history documenting a fall on the outstretched hand can be elicited. Presumably, such a fall produces a hyperextension strain across the midcarpal joint. For the scaphoid "link" to fail, it seems almost inevitable that this force must be sufficient to produce at least a transient subluxation of the joint. This is only one step away from the classic transscaphoid perilunate fracture dislocation that results from a more severe degree of trauma. Thus there must be a subtle difference between the degree of force required to produce a complete or unstable fracture of the scaphoid and that which produces an incomplete or stable fracture, in which the scaphoid has "hinged open" whilst maintaining some intact articular cartilage. It is somewhat academic to question the exact position of the wrist in which failure of the scaphoid occurs. However, since the line of the midcarpal joint crosses the proximal pole in radial deviation and the distal pole in ulnar deviation, it is tempting to postulate that the wrist deviation at the time of injury determines the line of the fracture. Mayfield[8] and Weber and Chao[9] have simulated scaphoid fractures in cadaver wrists, illustrating much about the mechanism of injury. However, major differences exist between living and cadaver wrists, and one may learn much about the mechanism of injury by correlating the patient's history with the findings at the time of surgery. For example, although it has been suggested that fractures of the scaphoid waist may occur by impingement of the scaphoid against the dorsal lip of the radius, I have found no evidence to support this hypothesis when operating on acute scaphoid fractures.

Thus, fractures of the *waist* are almost certainly the result of *shear* force across the bone. Fractures of the *tubercle* (Figure 2-8), like radial styloid fractures, appear to be caused by either *compression* or *avulsion*.[10] Associated fractures of the triquetrum also result from ligament avulsions. Similarly, it appears that extremely *small proximal pole* fractures may be caused by an *avulsion* of the attachment of the scapholunate ligament (Figure 2-9).

No doubt many fractures are the result of combined forces across the scaphoid (Figure 2-10), and an exact analysis of the mechanism of injury may not always be possible. For example, in theory a major hyperextension injury of the wrist may produce a scaphoid fracture or a scapholunate ligament rupture, but not both. For the scaphoid to fracture, one assumes that the ligament must remain intact and vice versa. Thus I was sceptical when a colleague told me that he had treated a patient in whom an unstable scaphoid fracture was associated with a complete rupture of the scapholunate ligament. Recently, I learned my lesson when I was asked to treat a patient with the same combination of injuries (Figure 2-11). After operating on this patient's wrist, I am still not certain exactly how this combination of injuries occurred. Presumably, the ligament rupture occurred either before or at the same time as the fracture, and one can only postulate a very subtle combination of major disruptive forces across the wrist.

Chapter 2

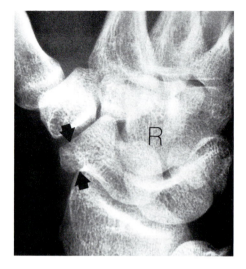

Figure 2-8. Fracture of the scaphoid tubercle. Although undisplaced, this fracture was probably caused by a *compression shearing* force (type IA).

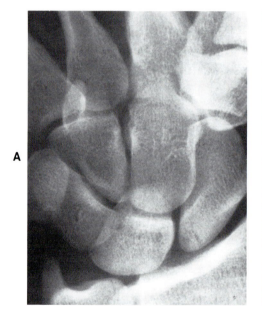
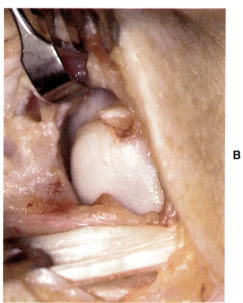

Figure 2-9. A, Radiograph of a small fracture through the proximal pole of the left scaphoid. **B,** Intraoperative photograph shows that this is an *avulsion* fracture associated with a scapholunate ligament injury.

Anatomy and Biomechanics

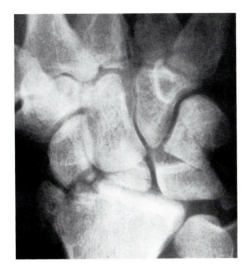

Figure 2-10. Radiograph of a patient who sustained severe trauma to the wrist. Apart from a transscaphoid-perilunate fracture dislocation (*shear strain*), there is also a *compression* fracture of the radius and an *avulsion* fracture of the ulnar styloid.

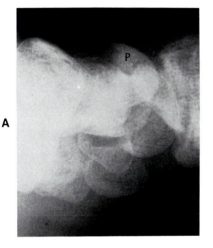

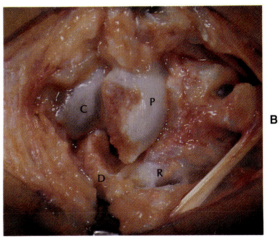

Figure 2-11. **A**, Lateral x-ray film at 6 weeks following closed treatment of a transscaphoid-perilunate fracture dislocation of the carpus. Note the position of the proximal pole (*PP*) of the scaphoid. **B**, Intraoperative photograph of patient shown in **A** (dorsal approach, right wrist). The proximal fragment (*P*) of the scaphoid was found to be dislocated dorsal to the radius (*R*) due to rupture of the scapholunate ligament. The distal pole (*D*) of the scaphoid and the capitate (*C*) were in normal position. Both fracture faces are seen clearly. Would you have noticed all this on the x-ray?

Chapter 2

Whatever the mechanism of injury, when treating a patient with a scaphoid fracture, it is important to remember that a radiograph seldom tells the whole story; certainly it can never reveal the true degree of joint and ligament damage that must almost inevitably accompany this injury (Figure 2-12). When looking at an x-ray film of a scaphoid fracture, try to make a three-dimensional picture of the bone in your mind. Remember how much force is required to break the scaphoid when you are deciding on treatment.

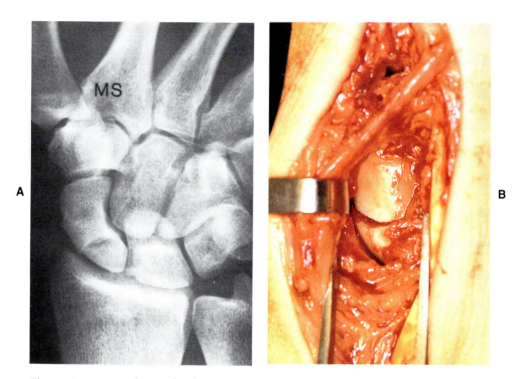

Figure 2-12. A, Radiograph of an acute scaphoid fracture. **B,** Intraoperative photograph of the same patient. Note the amount of bleeding into the soft tissues and the joint. The fracture is completely unstable and the articular cartilage has been damaged. These findings are not apparent on the x-ray film.

REFERENCES

1. Taleisnik J. Ligaments of the wrist. J Hand Surg 1:110, 1976.
2. Taleisnik J. The Wrist. Edinburgh: Churchill Livingstone, 1985.
3. Mayfield JK, Johnson RP, Kilcoyne RF. The ligaments of the human wrist and their functional significance. Anat Rec 186:417, 1976.
4. Gelberman RH, Panagis JS, Taleisnik J, Baumgartner M. The arterial anatomy of the human carpus. I. The extraosseous vascularities. J Hand Surg 8:367, 1983.
5. Panagis JS, Gelberman RH, Taleisnik J, Baumgartner M. The arterial anatomy of the human carpus. II. The intraosseous vascularities. J Hand Surg 8:375, 1983.
6. Gelberman RH, Menon J. The vascularity of the scaphoid bone. J Hand Surg 5:508, 1980.
7. Fisk E. Carpal instability in the fractured scaphoid. Ann R Coll Surg Engl 46:63, 1970.
8. Mayfield JK. Mechanism of carpal injuries. Clin Orthop 149:45, 1980.
9. Weber ER, Chao EY. Experimental approach to the mechanism of scaphoid waist fracture. J Hand Surg 3:142, 1978.
10. Prosser AJ, Brenkel IJ, Irvine GB. Articular fractures of the distal scaphoid. J Hand Surg 19B:87, 1988.

3

Diagnosis

The importance of obtaining an accurate
history cannot be overestimated because both
the treatment and the prognosis depend
on the type of fracture with which
one is dealing.

It is unfortunate that so much reliance is placed on the radiographical diagnosis of scaphoid fractures. The history and clinical examination are of equal importance; the patient who experiences pain and swelling of the wrist after a heavy fall on the outstretched hand has almost certainly sustained significant damage to the joint, even if the x-ray film appears quite normal. Whilst it is well known that the initial x-ray study may fail to demonstrate the presence of an acute scaphoid fracture, we tend to forget that radiographs give no indication as to the degree of damage to the soft tissue, ligaments, or articular cartilage that may have occurred at the time of injury (see Figure 2-12).

HISTORY OF INJURY

Approximately 90% of patients recall a hyperextension strain of the wrist after falling on their outstretched hand. It is rare for the patient to hear a "crack" unless the injury has been severe enough to produce a transscaphoid-perilunate fracture dislocation. Most patients are unable to recall whether the wrist was in radial or ulnar deviation at the time of impact. I have seldom seen grazing or bruising over the thenar or hypothenar eminences significant enough to help determine the direction of force applied to the wrist. However, I have the impression that a torsional force may be involved in some fractures; this may be confirmed at surgery, since displaced fractures often show evidence of rotary instability. Occasionally the patient insists that the wrist was in acute flexion at the moment of impact. It is hard to visualise how the scaphoid could be fractured in this position, and I have been unable to recognise any associated fracture pattern. However, I have learned to trust my patients and accept that we still do not fully understand the mechanism of fracture in this fascinating bone.

It is well known that 95% of patients with scaphoid fractures are males; the average age is approximately 25 years. However, this fracture is by no means uncommon in children as young as 8 years. I also have seen several women over 50 years of age with this injury.

Most fractures are the result of sporting injuries, particularly heavy falls when tackling during a game of football. Motorcycle accidents are another common cause of injury, with the fracture occurring either at the time of impact or a few moments later when the rider lands

Diagnosis

on the road. Fractures occurring at the time of impact are often severe, and it is not uncommon to see associated compression fractures of the distal radius. Extensive articular cartilage damage is often apparent at surgery (Figure 3-1). In general, fracture dislocations and proximal pole fractures tend to be associated with more severe degrees of trauma. In contrast, scaphoid fractures in women and children typically result from simple falls and relatively minor trauma.

The importance of obtaining an accurate history cannot be overestimated because both the treatment and the prognosis depend on the type of fracture with which one is dealing.

When the history is being obtained, it is extremely important to inquire about previous trauma, particularly if the patient does not relate the classic story of a recent injury. These patients may have a longstanding scaphoid fracture as a result of previous trauma of which they may or may not be aware. In many countries it is convenient to claim

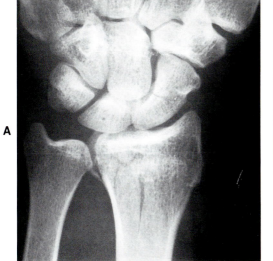
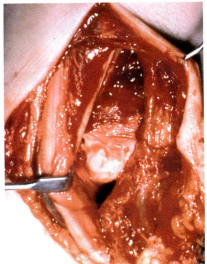

Figure 3-1. A, Radiograph of the wrist of a patient involved in a motorcycle accident. Note the transverse fracture of the scaphoid waist and the comminuted fracture involving the distal articular surface of the radius. **B,** Intraoperative findings; note the degree of bleeding in the soft tissues and the damage to the articular cartilage over the proximal pole of the scaphoid.

that a scaphoid fracture is the result of a recent work injury, but in my experience this is uncommon. I am convinced, however, that a second injury, sometimes relatively trivial, may be sufficient to convert an asymptomatic nonunion into a symptomatic one. (The mechanism for this is discussed in Chapter 4.)

EXAMINATION

Unfortunately for the patient, scaphoid fractures involve the dominant wrist more commonly than the nondominant one. Fortunately for the surgeon, however, there is normally an uninjured wrist with which the injured one may be compared. Bilateral fractures are rare (the incidence is approximately 2%), and these tend to have the worst prognosis.

Swelling may be gross or subtle but is always apparent when the anatomical snuff-box is examined in profile. Haemarthrosis is common in acute fractures, although seldom is there any visible bruising of the skin.

In the case of a transscaphoid-perilunate fracture dislocation, swelling may be extreme, with bleeding extending from the carpal tunnel into the forearm, producing an acute compartmental syndrome (Figure 3-2). The swelling may also involve the fascial compartments of the hand, and in this type of injury it is essential to check the intrinsic muscles for signs of impending ischaemia.

Dorsal swelling associated with an ununited fracture suggests chronic synovitis, which is a poor prognostic sign, indicative of avascular necrosis. Patients with long-standing scaphoid pseudarthrosis commonly display bony swelling on the back of the wrist due to dorsal osteophyte formation.

Tenderness, always present on deep palpation within the anatomical snuff-box, should localise the injury site to the scaphoid. Fractures of the tubercle are maximally tender on the volar surface at the base of the thumb, whereas proximal pole fractures may be palpated over the dorsum of the fully flexed wrist. Tenderness over the ulnar side of the wrist is common, particularly in acute injuries, and usually signifies midcarpal ligament injury or a dorsal avulsion fracture of the triquetrum.

Range of motion, especially extension, is normally restricted in patients with a scaphoid fracture. With acute injuries, all movements are restricted because of the pain associated with haemarthrosis.

In contrast, patients with established nonunion only experience pain at the extremes of motion, particularly when the wrist is forced into extension. Loss of wrist extension is pathognomonic of an ununited scaphoid fracture and is the result of the associated carpal collapse deformity and volar capsular contracture. In extreme cases extension may be lost completely. Deformity of the scaphoid also reduces the range of ulnar and radial deviation by up to 50%; a painful block to radial deviation is a symptom of the radiocarpal impingement syndrome caused by localised osteoarthritis. Occasionally a patient with an established non-

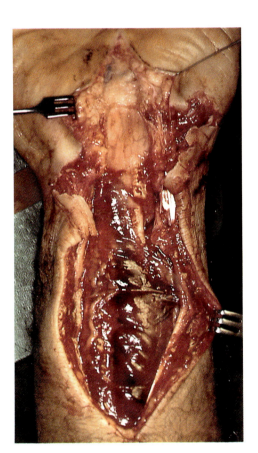

Figure 3-2. This patient presented with an acute fracture dislocation of the carpus, complicated by a closed compartmental syndrome affecting the distal forearm. Note the extensive haematoma; the median nerve has been decompressed by division of the flexor retinaculum.

union experiences painful restriction of wrist motion in all directions—the so-called irritable wrist. This painful restriction indicates chronic synovitis, which is a poor prognostic sign associated with avascular necrosis of the bone.

Abnormal mobility or clinically demonstrable carpal instability is seldom present except in patients with an acute unstable fracture dislocation; attempts to demonstrate this sign in such cases are unwise and unnecessary.

A stable, painless wrist is essential for satisfactory hand function. Since the scaphoid bone is the keystone of the wrist, patients with scaphoid injuries nearly always demonstrate some degree of functional disability. Measurement of the grip strength is a good indicator of hand function. A simple and reasonably accurate way of measuring grip strength is to ask the patient to grasp the examiner's middle and index fingers in both hands at the same time and to squeeze tightly. However, a Jamar dynamometer is de rigueur if published studies are contemplated. I have found measurement of grip strength to be an accurate indicator of healing after reconstructive surgery for scaphoid nonunion. Preoperatively, grip strength is commonly reduced by more than 50%, improves steadily after surgery, and returns to normal within 12 months.

RADIOGRAPHICAL EXAMINATION

As pointed out earlier, radiographs of the scaphoid never tell the whole story. Recalling that the scaphoid is a three-dimensional bone that lies at approximately 45 degrees to the long axis of the limb helps explain why radiographs may fail to show the true status of a scaphoid fracture. *The single most important x-ray film is the comparative view of the opposite uninjured wrist.*

Almost all the information needed can be obtained from high-quality plain x-ray films using the four standard views of the scaphoid (Figure 3-3).

Diagnosis

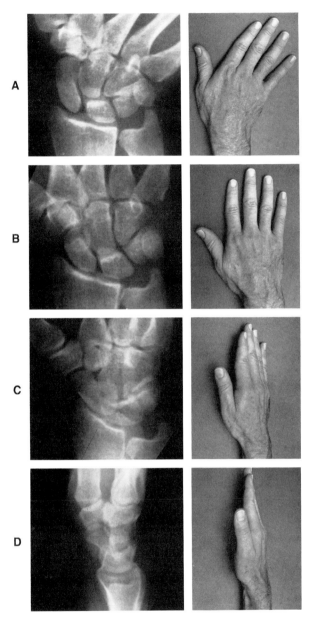

Figure 3-3. Four standard x-ray views of the wrist. **A**, Posteroanterior (PA) view with the wrist in full *ulnar deviation*. **B**, PA view with the wrist in full *radial deviation*. **C**, Forty-five degree oblique view. **D**, Lateral view with the wrist in a neutral position.

Chapter 3

Since the scaphoid flexes in radial deviation and extends in ulnar deviation (see Figure 3-3, *A-B*), the *length* of the bone should be assessed by comparing the *ulnar and radial deviation views* in *both wrists*. Assuming that the two views are identical, any difference in length must indicate a scaphoid deformity resulting from either a fracture or ligament injury (Figure 3-4). In *radial deviation,* an unstable fracture angulates forward (Figure 3-5), producing obvious shortening when compared to the opposite side. The *45-degree oblique view* may reveal a fracture not apparent on the posteroanterior films. This view may also demonstrate the displacement associated with unstable distal oblique fractures (Figure 3-6).

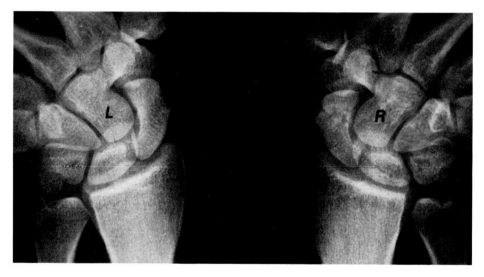

Figure 3-4. X-ray film of both wrists in ulnar deviation. The deformity associated with fracture of the right scaphoid is best appreciated by comparing it with the opposite uninjured side.

Diagnosis

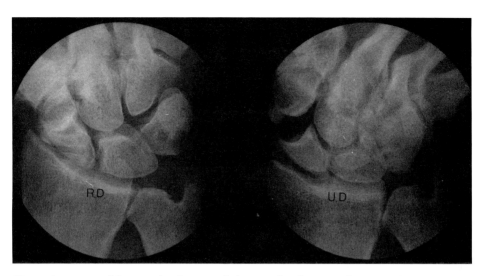

Figure 3-5. Unstable pseudarthrosis of the scaphoid. Note that in radial deviation (*RD*) the distal fragment has angulated forwards to the extent that the fracture line is no longer visible. *UD,* Ulnar deviation.

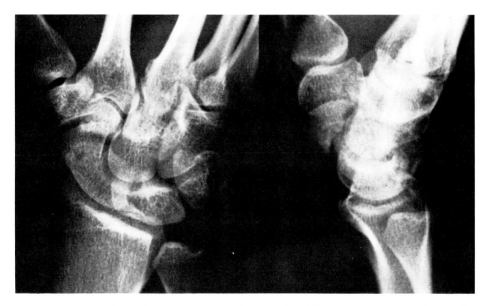

Figure 3-6. Note how displacement of this scaphoid fracture appears only on the semioblique view on the right; in the plain view on the left no displacement is evident.

Chapter 3

It is often difficult to define the scaphoid on the *lateral film*; the acute fracture is hard to see unless there is a transscaphoid-perilunate fracture dislocation, which is best appreciated in this view (Figure 3-7). The main value of the lateral x-ray examination is to demonstrate the overall alignment of the carpus. The distal articular surface of the lunate should be approximately perpendicular to the long axis of both the capitate and the radius; a dorsally tilted lunate is classified as a *dorsiflexion deformity* (the DISI pattern). This is seen only rarely in acute fractures and indicates gross carpal instability (Figure 3-8). It is more commonly seen in association with scaphoid pseudarthrosis, where it indicates the degree of carpal collapse deformity that has occurred. In advanced cases the capitolunate joint becomes subluxated and may show signs of degenerative arthritis (Figure 3-9).

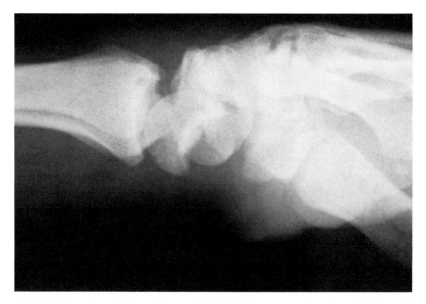

Figure 3-7. Dislocation of the midcarpal joint is best appreciated on the lateral x-ray film.

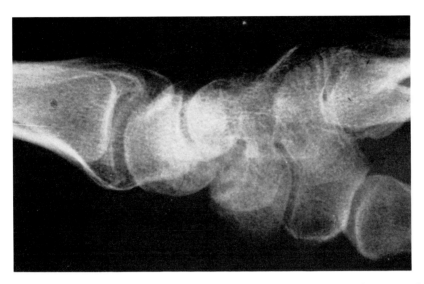

Figure 3-8. Lateral x-ray film of a patient with an acute unstable fracture of the scaphoid; note the associated dorsiflexion deformity (DISI) of the lunate.

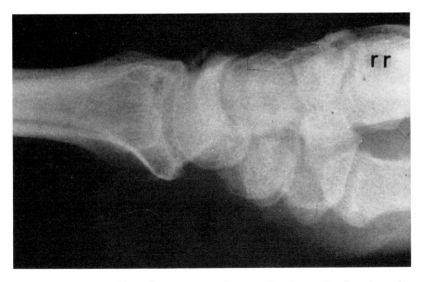

Figure 3-9. Lateral x-ray film of a patient with a scaphoid pseudarthrosis and associated carpal collapse deformity; note dorsiflexion deformity of the lunate with subluxation of the capitolunate joint leading to early degenerative arthritis.

If the distal articular surface of the lunate is angulated forwards, this indicates an unusual type of carpal instability (the volar intercalated segment instability or VISI pattern). This type of instability is seen only rarely in patients with scaphoid fractures and indicates disruption of the ulnar carpal ligaments.

I have not found it necessary to obtain stress x-rays of the scaphoid, although colleagues have told me that instability in an acute fracture of the scaphoid may be demonstrated by applying a radial distraction force to the wrist whilst the film is being taken. Stress cineradiography also may be used as a means of demonstrating instability of the scaphoid.

OTHER IMAGING TECHNIQUES

I do not believe that arthrography has any place in the diagnosis and management of acute or ununited scaphoid fractures. Although this imaging technique may demonstrate ruptures of the scapholunate ligament, the diagnosis can usually be made from the plain films. Arthrograms may give both false-positive and false-negative results.[1]

Nakamura et al.[2] have recently reported on the use of three-dimensional computed tomography as a method of demonstrating carpal displacements. This appears to be a useful technique.

Bone scans aid in the diagnosis of wrist pain. However, the findings are nonspecific, and minor joint damage or synovitis may give a positive result. If a scaphoid fracture is suspected but cannot be demonstrated radiographically, a bone scan confirms or excludes the presence of a significant bony injury. Some authors[3] claim that the bone scan can be used to assist in the diagnosis of avascular necrosis. However, I have never found the films to be of sufficient quality to differentiate clearly between the two halves of the scaphoid; in the presence of a fracture, an intense uptake of isotope throughout the radiocarpal joint normally occurs (Figure 3-10).

Diagnosis

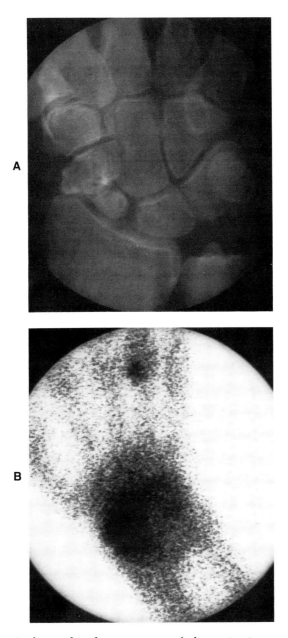

Figure 3-10. A, Radiographical appearance of the wrist in a patient with longstanding pseudarthrosis of the scaphoid and avascular necrosis of the proximal pole. **B,** Bone scan film of the same patient; note the generalised increased uptake on the radial side of the wrist. It is not possible to differentiate between the two fragments of the scaphoid.

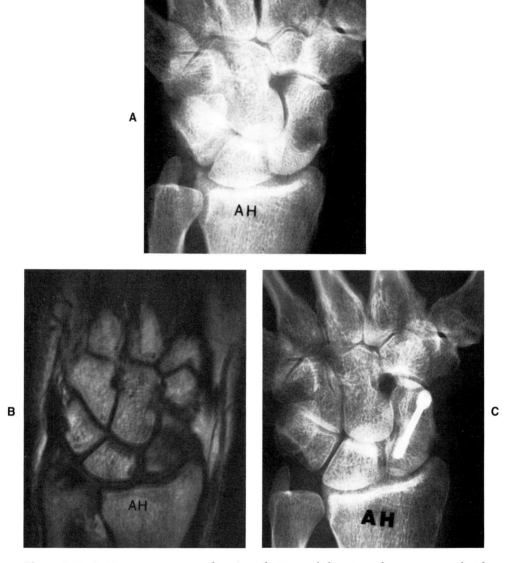

Figure 3-11. A, X-ray appearance after 6 weeks' immobilisation of an acute scaphoid fracture. The degree of cystic change and the speed of onset suggest that the proximal pole may be undergoing early avascular necrosis. **B,** *Magnetic resonance imaging* suggests that the bone in the proximal fragment is still viable. **C,** This patient was treated by bone grafting and internal fixation and the fracture healed uneventfully.

Magnetic resonance imaging may well be the best method of demonstrating the vascular status of the scaphoid (Figure 3-11). However, it is an expensive investigation, and its clinical significance has not yet been established.

REFERENCES
1. Herbert TJ, Faithfull RG, McCann DJ, Ireland J. Bilateral arthrography of the wrist. J Hand Surg 15B:233, 1990.
2. Nakamura R, Horii E, Tanaka Y, Imaeda T, Hayakawa N. Three-dimensional CT imaging for wrist disorders. J Hand Surg 14B:53, 1989.
3. Nielson PT, Hedeboe J, Thommesen P. Bone scintigraphy in the evaluation of fractures of the carpal scaphoid bone. Acta Orthop Scand 54:303, 1983.

4

Natural History

Nothing is more depressing than having
to fuse the wrist of a young patient who, a few
years earlier, suffered a simple fracture
of the scaphoid bone.

Chapter 4

Much is yet to be learned about the natural history of the acute scaphoid fracture. Some patients may have a scaphoid fracture without ever being aware of it, and not all of these patients develop symptoms in later life. At the other extreme are those patients who develop pseudarthrosis within a few months of injury despite prompt diagnosis and treatment of the acute fracture (Figure 4-1). Some patients may present with a pseudarthrosis years after the original fracture was believed to be soundly healed (Figure 4-2). Conversely, I have seen the occasional case where an obvious scaphoid fracture appears to have healed spontaneously without any form of treatment. How can such erratic behaviour be explained?

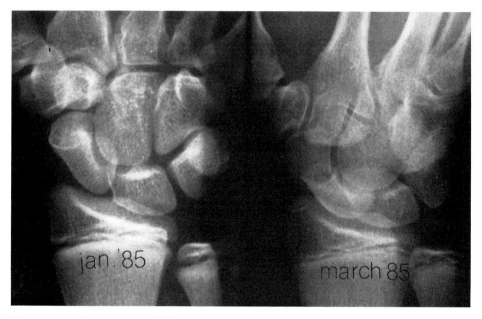

Figure 4-1. This 15-year-old boy sustained an acute scaphoid fracture in January 1985. The initial x-ray film showed no obvious fracture. However, despite prompt immobilisation of the wrist, x-ray films taken at the time of cast removal 6 weeks later showed the development of a pseudarthrosis with associated carpal instability. (From Herbert TJ. Scaphoid fractures: Operative treatment. In Barton NJ, ed. Fractures of the Hand and Wrist. Edinburgh: Churchill Livingstone, 1988, p 221.)

Natural History

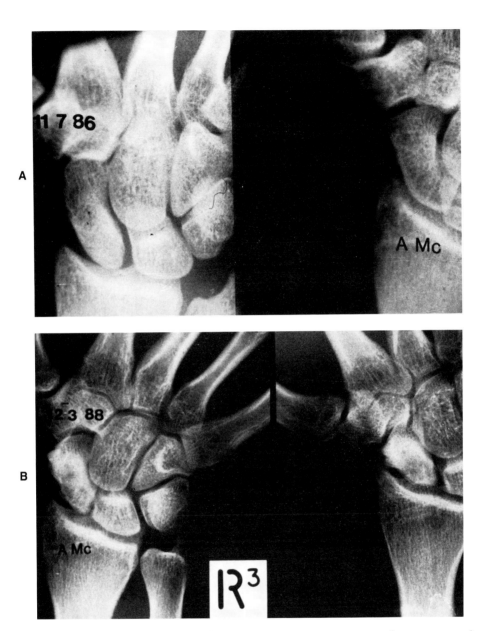

Figure 4-2. **A,** X-ray appearance following conservative treatment of an acute scaphoid fracture. Union appears complete. **B,** The patient returned 2 years later, at which time x-ray films showed marked deformity of the scaphoid associated with an unstable pseudarthrosis and possible avascular necrosis.

Chapter 4

I suspect the clue lies in the fact that the scaphoid is an intra-articular bone. In many ways scaphoid fractures behave similarly to subcapital fractures of the femoral neck; stable fractures tend to have a good prognosis, whereas unstable fractures have a high incidence of delayed union and late avascular necrosis. As a medical student I was taught that one of the causes of fracture nonunion was the effect of synovial fluid at the fracture site. Now that we tend to concentrate on the mechanical aspects of fractures, this concept is no longer in vogue, although I believe it may be relevant in the case of the scaphoid. This point was emphasised by Osterman[1] in his excellent review article on scaphoid nonunion. Certainly a common observation when operating on recent scaphoid fractures is the presence of a fold of synovium or capsule adherent to or actually trapped within the fracture site (Figure 4-3).

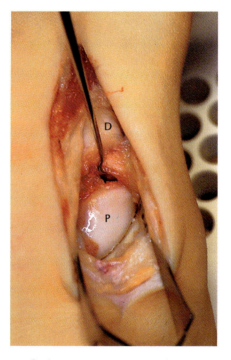

Figure 4-3. Intraoperative findings in a patient with delayed union of the scaphoid. Note the fold of capsule and synovium that was wedged between the fracture faces and is being lifted out with the small hook. *D,* Distal pole; *P,* proximal pole.

It has been suggested that the radioscaphocapitate ligament acts as a fulcrum over which the scaphoid may fracture. If this is the case, it is easy to see how this ligament may become trapped between the bone fragments, preventing accurate reduction and setting the scene for the development of fibrous union.[2] Even without soft tissue interposition at the fracture site, I believe that synovial adhesions and ingrowth, possibly combined with the effects of the synovial fluid itself, may result in fibrous as opposed to true osseous union. Perhaps this may be the body's own mechanism for stabilising intra-articular fractures, since it is clear that a firm fibrous union results in a stable scaphoid with few or no symptoms. However, the fibrous union renders the bone unduly susceptible to further trauma, leading to the development of an unstable nonunion.

It is often difficult to differentiate radiologically between fibrous and bony union. I believe this may explain why an apparently "healed" scaphoid fracture may present some years later as a pseudarthrosis.

If one accepts this hypothesis, then one must question the efficacy of closed treatment in the majority of patients with scaphoid fractures. For sound bone union to take place, the fracture faces must be in close apposition so that soft tissue interposition or synovial fluid cannot affect healing. These conditions would pertain in the case of an incomplete fracture, and we know that these have an excellent prognosis with minimal treatment. However, if closed treatment is used for complete fractures, then osseous union may be the result more of luck than skill.

What then is the natural history of the acute scaphoid fracture? Assuming good position of the bone fragments and immobilisation of the fracture, union should be well advanced by 6 weeks. However, if soft tissue interposition or synovial ingrowth occurs, the stage is set for the development of fibrous union. Whether this eventually progresses to osseous union is open to speculation. More likely, the fibrous union will eventually break down, leading to instability and the development of a true pseudarthrosis.

The excellent studies of Mack et al.[3] and Ruby, Stinson, and Belsky[4] have shown that the natural history of the unstable scaphoid pseudarthrosis is one of progressive collapse deformity followed by radiocarpal osteoarthritis. Over time, bone wear at the fracture site leads to marked shortening of the scaphoid and an obvious discrepancy in the

Chapter 4

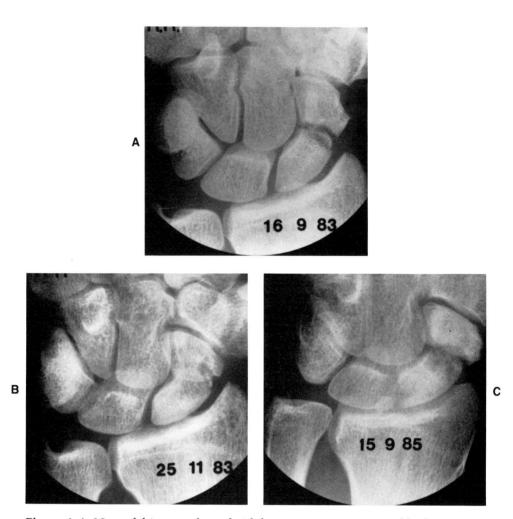

Figure 4-4. Natural history of scaphoid fracture. **A,** Acute unstable fracture. **B,** Carpal collapse deformity is apparent following 2 months of cast immobilisation. **C,** Two years later there is an established pseudarthrosis; note size discrepancy between the two fragments and early osteoarthritic changes.

size of the two fragments (Figure 4-4). Impingement between the palmar flexed distal pole of the scaphoid and the styloid process of the radius results in radiocarpal osteoarthritis. At the same time, the unsupported carpus collapses, with increasing subluxation and secondary arthritis of the midcarpal joint. As shown by Watson and Ryu,[5] the articulations between the proximal pole of the scaphoid, lunate, and radius remain relatively unaffected.

I have observed that the amount of carpal collapse deformity determines the extent to which wrist extension is limited, although the degree depends on the laxity of the patient's joints. If loss of wrist extension is significant, the patient experiences pain whenever the hand is forced backwards; this is the main cause of functional disability in patients with established nonunion. In time, particularly with increasing radiocarpal and midcarpal osteoarthritis, wrist motion becomes restricted to the extent that reconstructive surgery is no longer feasible and fusion becomes the best solution.

Nothing is more depressing than having to fuse the wrist of a young patient who, a few years earlier, suffered a simple fracture of the scaphoid bone. Unfortunately, this is an operation that I am still obliged to carry out several times a year. I believe that fusion of the wrist can be avoided, provided a more aggressive approach is taken towards the treatment of the acute scaphoid fracture.

REFERENCES

1. Osterman AL, Mikulics M. Scaphoid nonunion. Hand Clin 4(3):437, 1988.
2. Wilton TJ. Soft tissue interposition as a possible cause of scaphoid non-union. J Hand Surg 12B:50, 1987.
3. Mack GR, Bosse MJ, Gelberman RH, Yu E. The natural history of scaphoid nonunion. J Bone Joint Surg 66A:504, 1984.
4. Ruby LK, Stinson J, Belsky MR. The natural history of scaphoid nonunion: A review of fifty-five cases. J Bone Joint Surg 67A:428, 1985.
5. Watson HK, Ryu J. Degenerative disorders of the carpus. Orthop Clin North Am 15(2):337, 1984.

5

A Rational Approach to Treatment of Acute Scaphoid Fractures

> ... We must seriously question the routine use of plaster casting in the treatment of these injuries. ... It therefore behoves us to determine at the outset what type of fracture we are treating.

Chapter 5

Once we accept that fractures of the scaphoid, like other intra-articular fractures, have a significant complication rate, then we must seriously question the routine use of plaster casting in the treatment of these injuries. Whilst this treatment modality may be adequate for *stable fractures*, it seldom is for *unstable fractures*. It therefore behoves us to determine at the outset what type of fracture we are treating. A classification system based on the x-ray appearance of the acute fracture has proved useful in differentiating fracture types and determining the best method of management (see pp. 62 to 66).

STABLE FRACTURES

In the case of stable, or incomplete, fractures of the scaphoid, reduction is unnecessary. If the fracture is sufficiently protected to prevent it from becoming unstable, union should occur rapidly, with little or no risk of complications.[1] The wrist may be protected by immobilisation in a short-arm Colles'-type cast for approximately 6 weeks. Experience has shown that it is unnecessary to incorporate the base of the thumb in the cast for stable fractures. This makes the treatment much more acceptable to the patient, since leaving the thumb out of the cast means that most manual tasks can be performed without difficulty (Figure 5-1, *A* and *B*).

Unfortunately, it is not always easy to decide whether the fracture is stable or not. We have already seen how the initial x-ray appearance may be deceptive (Chapter 1). However, despite adequate immobilisation, subsequent films may show signs of increasing displacement and deformity, indicating instability (Figure 5-2).

Therefore we must learn *never* to trust the x-ray film. In doubtful cases it is reasonable to give a trial period of immobilisation in a short-arm cast, provided the patient agrees. Adequate follow-up is essential, since subsequent x-ray examinations may reveal problems that were not apparent on the original films. I normally remove the cast after 1 month and encourage the patient to exercise the wrist, regardless of the clinical or radiological findings.

Should the fracture appear to be healing, further immobilisation is unnecessary, although the patient is advised to protect the wrist from trauma until 3 months from the time of injury. As with other fractures

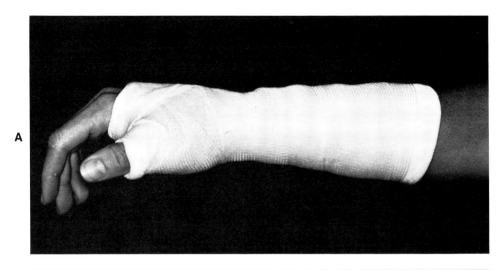

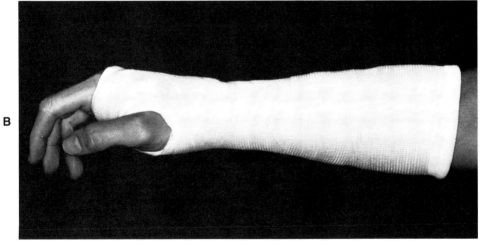

Figure 5-1. Methods of splinting for management of scaphoid fractures. **A,** Standard scaphoid cast that includes the base of the thumb. The author no longer uses this type of cast. **B,** Colles'-type cast, with the thumb free, causes less restriction on hand function. By immobilising the midcarpal joint, this provides sufficient protection for stable scaphoid fractures. (Courtesy Paul R. Manske, M.D.)

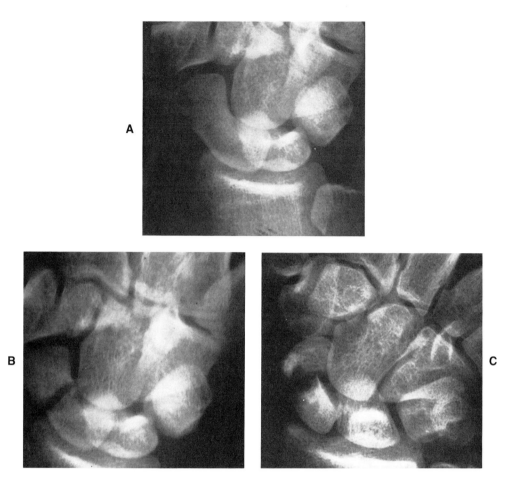

Figure 5-2. Radiographical series showing progressive deterioration of a scaphoid fracture treated by immobilisation in a plaster cast. The patient was a 21-year-old man who had fallen on his outstretched hand. **A,** X-ray appearance at the time of initial examination. The fracture is hard to see and was considered to be stable. **B,** X-ray appearance after 6 weeks' immobilisation in a scaphoid cast. Note that there are now signs of instability. **C,** X-ray appearance at 6 months; there is now a well-established unstable pseudarthrosis.

around the wrist, a stable fracture should be united within 4 to 6 weeks but may not be consolidated for up to 3 months. Careful follow-up of these patients is essential; I recommend clinical and radiological examination at 6-week intervals until the outcome is clear. I ask all patients to return for review after 1 year, although I must confess that patient compliance is not always ideal. However, I have found that most patients are prepared to cooperate once they understand that their treatment is designed to avoid lengthy periods in plaster casts.

Alternatively, if signs of (fracture) displacement or of a developing nonunion (Figure 5-3) appear, then the patient is advised to undergo internal fixation. Surgery is delayed for 2 to 3 weeks, allowing sufficient time to reverse the osteoporosis that inevitably occurs during the period in plaster casting.

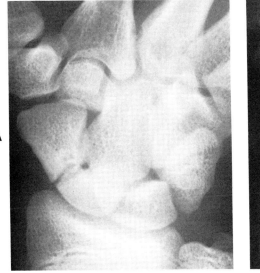
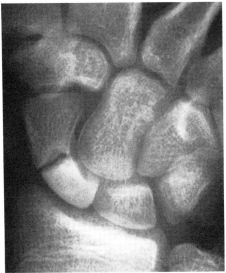

Figure 5-3. A, X-ray film showing an acute unstable fracture through the waist of the scaphoid in a 16-year-old boy. **B,** X-ray appearance following immobilisation in plaster for 6 weeks. Note the relative density of the proximal pole fragment in contrast to the surrounding osteoporosis. The bone was found to be healthy at surgery, and the fracture went on to sound union. *It is incorrect to call this finding avascular necrosis* (see Chapter 8).

Chapter 5

"CLINICAL" FRACTURES

If the initial x-ray examination fails to demonstrate a fracture, even though the history and clinical signs suggest this diagnosis, the same treatment regimen as for stable fractures is used, provided that one can confidently exclude a diagnosis of rotary dislocation of the scaphoid. It is not always easy to differentiate between ligament injury and an occult fracture. A high level of awareness and careful clinical and radiological assessment at regular intervals are required. Ligament injuries are discussed in Chapter 12. If a fracture is suspected, the scaphoid should be reexamined both clinically and radiologically (out of plaster) after 2 weeks. When doubts about the diagnosis remain, a bone scan may be used to confirm or exclude the presence of a fracture.

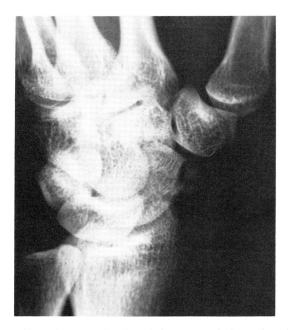

Figure 5-4. X-ray film shows a displaced fracture of the tubercle involving the scaphotrapezial joint. It is unnecessary to reduce or immobilise this fracture.

TUBERCLE FRACTURES

Fractures of the tubercle tend to be relatively benign injuries. Quite commonly, a bone fragment from the tubercle appears displaced, suggesting an avulsion injury (Figure 5-4). Although the fracture normally involves the scaphotrapezial joint, it is probably unnecessary to try to reduce or immobilise the fracture. I treat tubercle fractures as soft tissue injuries. The wrist is splinted only until the acute reaction has settled. After the splinting period, a short course of physiotherapy normally accelerates recovery. Although x-ray films commonly show persistent displacement and fibrous union of the fracture, this finding seldom causes disability. Occasionally I have seen patients with persistent pain and stiffness of the scaphotrapezial joint after a tubercle fracture. Such symptoms should respond to manipulation and steroid injection of the scaphotrapezial joint. However, on two occasions I have been forced to explore the joint and remove the loose fragment. Interestingly, both these patients had been treated by prolonged immobilisation in plaster casts because x-ray films had shown signs of delayed union. As with other avulsion fractures, I believe it is better to ignore the x-ray appearance and treat the soft tissue injury.

UNSTABLE FRACTURES (TYPE B)

If the initial x-ray examination shows a complete fracture, the chances are the fracture is unstable and carries a high risk of complications. Although displacement is generally accepted as a sign of instability, this is not always apparent on plain x-ray examination; I have learned to suspect any fracture that involves both cortices of the bone.

Proximal pole fractures (type B3) are always complete and seldom, if ever, heal without surgery (Figure 5-5). Similarly, distal oblique fractures (type B1) and fracture dislocations (type B4) are always complete and should therefore be classified as unstable (see pp. 63-64).

Chapter 5

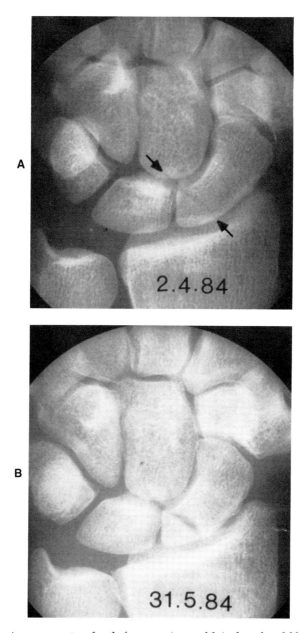

Figure 5-5. A, Acute *proximal pole* fracture (unstable); this should have been treated by internal fixation. **B,** Nonunion is inevitable following conservative treatment, as shown here.

Retrospective studies have shown that unstable fractures have a high incidence of complications with conservative treatment. Since 1977 I have routinely treated all type B, or unstable, fractures by primary open reduction and internal fixation. The results[1] appear to justify this aggressive approach. Operating on these acute fractures, I have learned for myself lessons so clearly outlined by McLaughlin[2] more than 30 years ago. A considerable amount of blood usually pools in the joint, and the degree of damage to the soft tissues and articular cartilage is always greater than one would suspect from the x-ray appearance (Figure 5-6). The fracture is often so unstable that accurate reduction can be extremely difficult to achieve; one often wonders how conservative treatment of such fractures can ever produce satisfactory results.

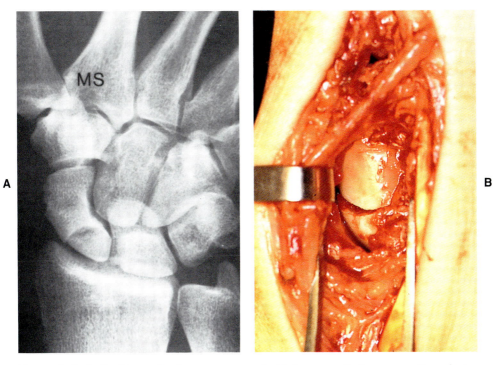

Figure 5-6. A, Radiograph of an acute scaphoid fracture. **B,** Intraoperative photograph of the same patient. Note the amount of bleeding into the soft tissues and the joint. The fracture is completely unstable and the articular cartilage has been damaged. These findings are not apparent on the x-ray film.

Chapter 5

The surgical technique for open reduction and internal fixation of the scaphoid is detailed in Chapter 6. The same principles apply as for all intra-articular fractures:
1. Accurate anatomical reduction
2. Atraumatic surgical technique
3. Rigid internal fixation
4. Repair of soft tissues and joint stabilisation
5. Early postoperative joint mobilisation

Although these principles are known to produce the best results in patients with other intra-articular fractures, many surgeons still have difficulty applying them to fractures of the carpal scaphoid and remain satisfied with the routine use of conservative treatment for all types of scaphoid fractures. Perhaps this hesitancy relates to the difficulty in achieving accurate anatomical reduction and rigid internal fixation and the expertise that this type of surgery demands. Furthermore, it is argued that this approach may subject the patient to unnecessary surgery.

Whilst I would not urge anyone to change a method of treatment that they have found satisfactory, I would caution against complacency and will continue to challenge published results on conservative treatment unless these have adequate and long-term follow-up. Only recently has any effort been made to review the late results after conservative treatment[3]; the indications are that nonunion is far more frequent than previous teachings would have us believe.

Another force for change must be reckoned with . . . the patient. The most important lesson that I have learned from patients with scaphoid fractures is that they do not like the standard scaphoid cast. Many will only tolerate casting for a few weeks and must be convinced that the outcome is likely to be a normal wrist. Given the choice between treatment in a cast or primary internal fixation with early functional recovery, many patients opt for the latter, particularly when their livelihood depends on the use of their hands.

Which one would you choose? Of course, you would want to know more about the operative procedure. You would only opt for surgery if you knew that the procedure were a relatively minor one, with predictable results and a low complication rate. You would then weigh the advantages and disadvantages of both methods of treatment before making your decision.

Having had the opportunity to carry out this exercise on many occasions, I now have no hesitation in recommending open reduction and internal fixation as the treatment of choice for acute, unstable fractures of the scaphoid. A rational approach to the management of acute scaphoid fractures is summarised below (Figure 5-7).

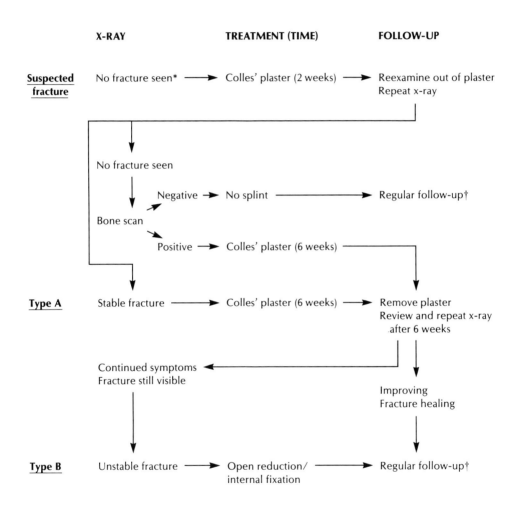

*Essential to exclude acute scapholunate ligament tear by appropriate investigations. (See Chapter 12.)
†All patients should be reviewed with new x-rays at 1 year.

Figure 5-7. A rational approach to treatment of the acute scaphoid fracture.

Chapter 5

Classification of Scaphoid Fractures*

TYPE A: STABLE ACUTE FRACTURES

Features:
- Fracture appears incomplete (only one cortex involved)
- Union normally rapid
- Minimal treatment required

Type A1: Fracture of Tubercle

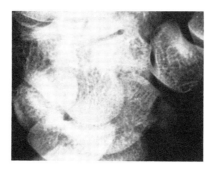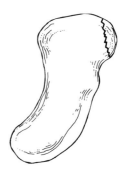

Type A2: Incomplete Fracture Through Waist

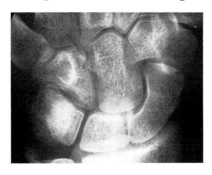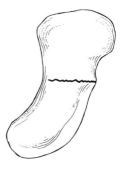

NOTE: It is sometimes difficult to determine on the initial x-ray examination whether or not the fracture is stable. Apart from fractures of the tubercle, it is essential to repeat the x-ray examination (out of the plaster cast) after 2 to 3 weeks.

---

*This classification is based on the radiological appearance of the fracture. It has been used since 1977 and has proved useful in the management of all types of scaphoid fractures. (Modified from Herbert TJ, Fisher WE. Management of the fractured scaphoid using a new bone screw. J Bone Joint Surg 66B:114-123, 1984.)

TYPE B: UNSTABLE ACUTE FRACTURES

Features:
- Fracture likely to displace in plaster
- Delayed union common
- Internal fixation is the treatment of choice

Type B1: Distal Oblique Fracture

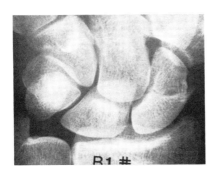 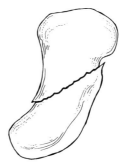

NOTE: Displacement in this type of fracture is often best seen on the 45-degree oblique film.

Type B2: Complete Fracture of Waist

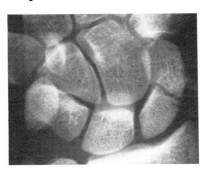 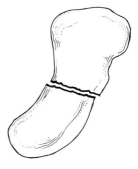

NOTE: Displacement is not always apparent, even when the fracture is unstable. Any fracture line that crosses both cortices is almost certainly unstable.

Chapter 5

Type B3: Proximal Pole Fracture

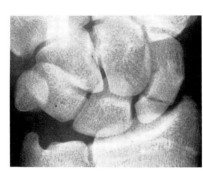 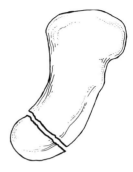

NOTE: Proximal pole fractures are always unstable, even though they may be difficult to see on the initial x-ray examination.

Type B4: Transscaphoid-Perilunate Fracture Dislocation of Carpus

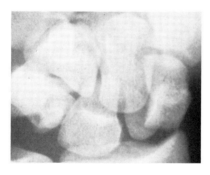 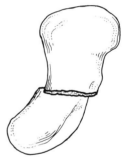

NOTE: The midcarpal dislocation is best appreciated on lateral films. Associated fractures of the triquetrum are common.

TYPE C: DELAYED UNION

Features:
- Widening of the fracture line
- Development of cysts adjacent to the fracture
- Relative density of the proximal fragment

Type C: Delayed Union

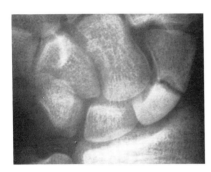
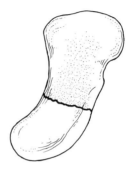

NOTE: Osteoporosis with relative density of proximal fragment—a common finding after immobilisation in plaster.

Chapter 5

TYPE D: ESTABLISHED NONUNION

Type D1: Fibrous Union

Features:
- Common after conservative treatment
- Relatively stable
- Little or no deformity
- Variable cystic change
- Likely to progress to pseudarthrosis in time
- Surgery is normally required

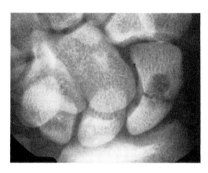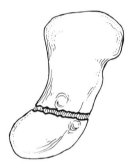

NOTE: Widening of fracture line with cystic change but no deformity or instability.

Type D2: Pseudarthrosis

Features:
- Usually unstable
- Progressive deformity
- Leads to development of osteoarthritis
- May result following untreated fibrous union (type D1)
- Surgery is normally required

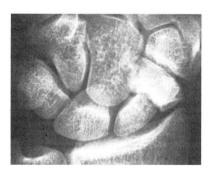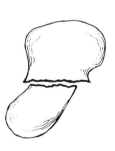

NOTE: Shortening, deformity, and discrepancy between size of bone fragments.

REFERENCES

1. O'Brien L, Herbert TJ. Internal fixation of acute scaphoid fractures: A new approach to treatment. Aust NZ J Surg 55:387, 1985.
2. McLaughlin HL. Fractures of the carpal navicular (scaphoid) bone: Some observations based on treatment by open reduction and internal fixation. J Bone Joint Surg 36A:763, 1954.
3. Dias JJ, Brenkel IJ, Finlay DBL. Patterns of union in fractures of the waist of the scaphoid. J Bone Joint Surg 71B:307, 1989.

6

Acute Fractures and Delayed Union
Surgical Techniques

The aim of treatment is to achieve accurate articular apposition of the two fragments, taking care that they are correctly aligned and that no malrotation exists.

Since the surgical techniques for acute scaphoid fractures and delayed unions are essentially the same, both will be covered in this chapter. The principles of surgery bear repeating:
1. Adequate exposure of the fracture(s).
2. Stable anatomical reduction with accurate realignment of the articular surfaces.
3. Sound internal fixation.
4. Careful repair of the soft tissues.
5. Early postoperative joint mobilisation.

SURGICAL APPROACHES TO THE SCAPHOID
Volar Approach (Figure 6-1)

Under normal circumstances, the best approach to the scaphoid is the standard volar incision, similar to that originally described by Russe.[1]

Make a curved skin incision* (Figure 6-1, A) just radial to the flexor carpi radialis (FCR) tendon, extending at least 3 cm proximally from the prominence of the scaphoid tubercle. The tubercle is best palpated with the wrist in radial deviation and lies at the base of the thenar eminence, immediately distal to the distal flexion crease of the wrist and just to the radial side of the FCR tendon.

Incise the sheath of the FCR tendon and retract the tendon in an ulnar direction (Figure 6-1, B). Beneath the tendon lies the volar capsule of the wrist, directly overlying the scaphoid bone. On the radial side lies the radial neurovascular bundle, which does not need to be exposed. However, the superficial palmar branch of the radial artery normally crosses towards the palm at the distal end of the incision. Unless it is unusually large (requiring mobilisation and preservation), ligate and divide this vessel to provide adequate access to the distal end of the scaphoid.

---

*Because of the tendency of this incision to produce keloid scars, particularly in females, a zig-zag incision may be preferred.

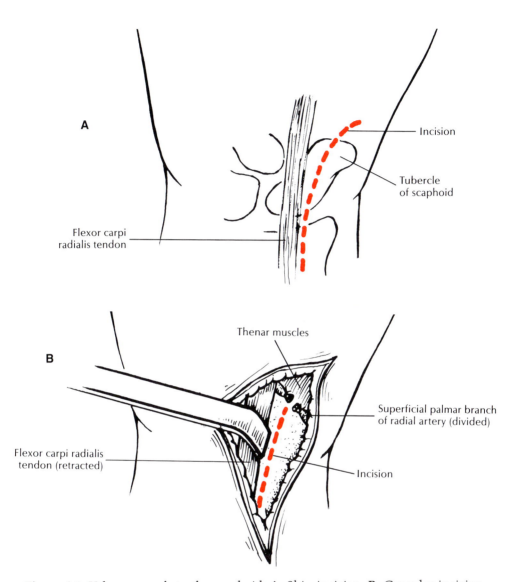

Figure 6-1. Volar approach to the scaphoid. **A,** Skin incision. **B,** Capsular incision. Note that the capsule is incised longitudinally along the line of the flexor carpi radialis tendon to expose the palmar surface of the scaphoid bone and the fracture. (**A-C** redrawn from Herbert TJ. Surgical Technique. The Herbert Bone Screw, rev. ed. Warsaw, Ind.: Zimmer, Inc., Technical Publication, 1987, p 10.)   *Continued.*

Chapter 6

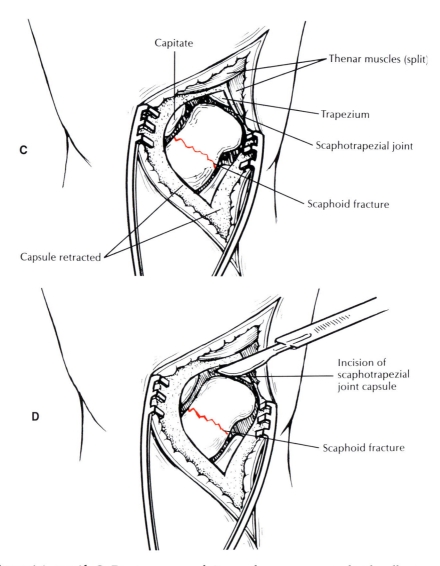

Figure 6-1, cont'd. C, Fracture exposed. It may be necessary to divide adhesions at the fracture site in order to obtain adequate visualisation. By moving the hand into ulnar and radial deviation, movement at the fracture site may be demonstrated, and by dorsiflexing the wrist, the fracture may be hinged open. In the case of fibrous union, the sharp end of the dissector may be required to prise open the fracture. **D,** Incision of capsule of the scaphotrapezial joint. The distal end of the scaphoid should be mobilised sufficiently to allow easy application of the scaphoid jig used for internal fixation. (**D** redrawn from Barton NJ, ed. Fractures of the Hand and Wrist. Edinburgh: Churchill Livingstone, 1988, p 230.)

Incise the capsule longitudinally throughout the length of the incision, taking care not to damage the underlying articular cartilage of the scaphoid. At the proximal end of the incision a condensation of the capsule (the radiolunate ligament) appears as a "labrum" to the radiocarpal joint. Divide the ligament to provide adequate exposure. Insertion of a small self-retaining retractor normally provides excellent visualisation of the entire volar surface of the scaphoid (Figure 6-1, *C*). However, if as a result of previous surgery significant scarring or soft tissue contractures have occurred, it may be necessary to elevate the capsule from the lip of the radius to obtain adequate exposure.

An acute fracture is usually accompanied by a haemarthrosis, which needs to be aspirated before the fracture can be visualised adequately. In the nonacute fracture, the synovium and capsule often adhere to the fracture site and need to be cleared for adequate exposure.

Carefully examine the scaphoid, assessing its size and shape, the degree of deformity, and the fracture itself. The proximal pole is best examined by distracting the wrist and passing a curved dissector around between the scaphoid and the radius. Identify the scapholunate ligament to obtain a clear picture of the width of the proximal pole. Similarly, define the medial border of the scaphoid at waist level either by palpation or by making a small incision in the capsule between the scaphoid and the capitate; the scaphoid waist is often remarkably narrow at this point. The radial and dorsal aspects of the bone also may be palpated using a curved dissector, although the soft tissue attachments along the spiral ridge prevent the dissector from being passed distally. Identify the scaphotrapezial joint distal to the scaphoid tubercle and open the joint if necessary (Figure 6-1, *D*). Mobilise the joint by carefully sweeping a small knife blade around the tubercle in a radial and then proximal direction, taking care not to damage the articular cartilage or to interfere with the blood supply where the soft tissues are attached to the distal end of the spiral groove. It is perfectly safe to dissect the soft tissues off the lateral border of the tubercle to a depth of at least 1 cm when mobilising the distal pole of the scaphoid.

Chapter 6

Extended Volar Approach

In the case of complex fracture dislocations of the wrist, an extended volar approach is required to gain adequate access to the carpus and to allow decompression of the carpal tunnel and of the forearm fascia if required. I prefer to use a lazy S–shaped incision, taking care to provide adequate access to the scaphotrapezial joint.

Dorsolateral Approach

A dorsolateral approach to the scaphoid has been recommended by Fisk[2] and others. However, access to the scaphoid is limited with this approach unless the radial styloid process is removed, which seems to add unnecessary complications to the procedure. Painful neuromas after retraction of the superficial branches of the radial nerve are common, and the radial artery is at risk as it passes dorsally across the distal end of the scaphoid. Furthermore, the soft tissue attachments to the spiral groove may be damaged when using this approach, placing the blood supply to the scaphoid at risk. For these reasons, I believe the dorsolateral approach has little to recommend it.

Dorsal Approach (Figure 6-2)

The proximal pole of the scaphoid and the scapholunate ligament are best exposed using a dorsal approach. Make a straight or curved skin incision over the back of the wrist, centred on the scapholunate junction, which is palpable in a small hollow just distal and ulnar to Lister's tubercle. Extend the incision for at least 2 cm distally and for a similar distance proximally from this point (Figure 6-2, *A*). Mobilise the extensor pollicis longus tendon by incising the extensor retinaculum over the third compartment and retract the tendon radially. Flex the wrist joint and incise the dorsal capsule longitudinally along the ulnar border of the extensor carpi radialis brevis tendon. Elevate the capsule from the lip of the radius to provide further exposure medially and laterally. This limited arthrotomy gives an excellent view of the entire proximal pole of the scaphoid, together with the scapholunate ligament (Figure 6-2, *B*). As with the volar approach, it is useful to define the medial border of the

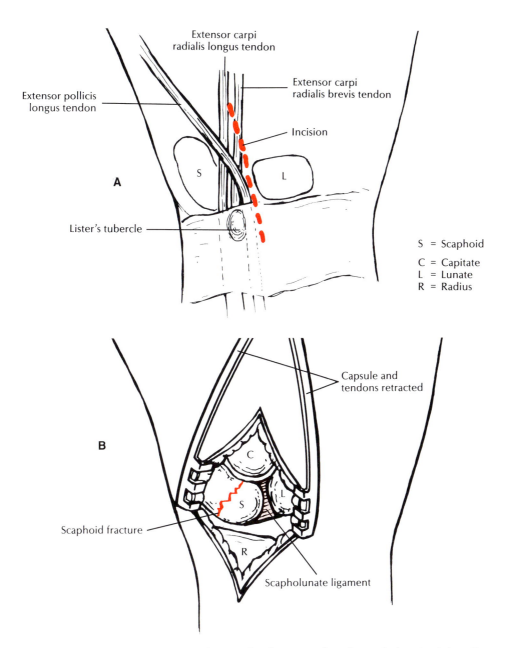

Figure 6-2. Dorsal approach to the scaphoid. **A,** Landmarks and skin incision. **B,** Capsule is incised to show proximal pole of scaphoid and scapholunate ligament.

scaphoid by making a small incision in the capsule between the scaphoid and the capitate. However, the important soft tissue attachments along the spiral groove must be carefully preserved, and the distal end of the scaphoid and the scaphotrapezial joint can only be exposed by making a separate distal incision in the capsule.

Extending the capsular incision in an ulnar direction will expose the capitate, lunate, or triquetrum should these bones or the dorsal capsule require repair. Although small proximal pole fractures may be accurately reduced using this approach, fractures of the waist and of the distal third of the scaphoid are not well visualised and are best treated using the anterior approach.

FRACTURE REDUCTION

Once the scaphoid has been exposed adequately and the haemarthrosis aspirated, carefully assess the fracture. Reposition or remove loose fragments of bone or articular cartilage and carry out a trial reduction. At this stage, it is important to remove any soft tissue trapped between the fracture faces; in the case of a developing nonunion, thoroughly curette fibrous cysts until the bone surfaces appear healthy.

After curettage or whenever significant bone loss or comminution has occurred, cancellous bone grafting should be carried out. The aim of treatment is to achieve accurate articular apposition of the two fragments, taking care that they are correctly aligned and that no malrotation exists. The fracture should be stable on compression; any tendency to collapse should be corrected by adequate bone grafting.

Once satisfactory reduction has been achieved, place a medium-sized Kirschner wire across the fracture. Insert the wire through the distal end of the tubercle towards the ulnar side of the bone and carefully pass the wire down the long axis of the bone, so that it crosses perpendicular to the fracture. To obtain adequate fixation, drill the wire into but not through the cortex of the proximal fragment.

At this stage, expose, reduce, and fix any associated fractures (e.g., radial styloid, triquetrum) as appropriate. If the midcarpal joint has been dislocated, check the reduction both visually and radiologically.

INTERNAL FIXATION

Whenever possible, rigid internal fixation should be achieved because it allows early postoperative joint mobilisation, which is one of the aims of surgery. The surgeon should use whatever method of internal fixation he or she finds satisfactory.

The simplest method is to place a second Kirschner wire towards the radial side of the scaphoid. However, this method is unlikely to give rigid fixation, and indeed the fracture surfaces may be distracted unless great care is taken during insertion of the wires (Figure 6-3). Postoperative plaster immobilisation is almost always required, as is a second procedure to remove the pins. Consequently, this method of fixation is not ideal and should only be employed if the fracture is not suitable for compression screw fixation.

I have no experience in the use of surgical staples for fixing scaphoid fractures, nor have results been published to date. The idea of

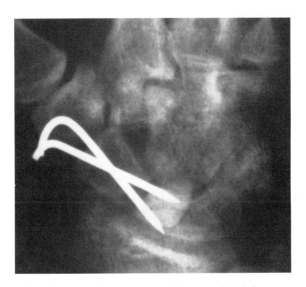

Figure 6-3. X-ray film showing distraction of the scaphoid fragments after internal fixation with excessively large, crossed Kirschner wires. It is clear that this fracture will not unite.

Chapter 6

staple fixation of the scaphoid does not appeal to me, since the implant must lie directly over the articular surface of the bone. Furthermore, it seems unlikely that rigid fixation could be achieved, and since the line of fixation is anterior to the long axis of the bone, there must be a real risk of volar collapse deformity occurring in the presence of comminuted or highly unstable fractures. The same objections apply to the use of the Ender plate, which requires supplementary plaster fixation and a second operation for removal of the implant.[3]

Intramedullary fixation using a compression screw is undoubtedly the best available method of fixing scaphoid fractures. I prefer the Herbert bone screw (Figure 6-4) to the standard type of cancellous or

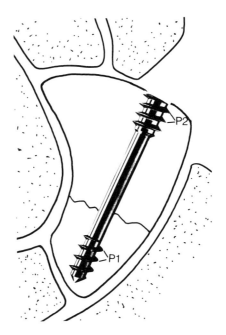

Figure 6-4. The Herbert bone screw, designed specifically for rigid internal fixation of scaphoid fractures. Features include: (1) double thread permitting fixation in both fragments; (2) pitch difference ($P1 > P2$) between the two threads producing compression; (3) absence of a conventional screw head allowing for insertion through joint surfaces; (4) threads designed to hold small osteochondral fragments; and (5) 4 mm diameter allowing optimal positioning in small bones. (From Herbert TJ. Use of the Herbert bone screw in surgery of the wrist. Clin Orthop 202:79, 1986.)

Acute Fractures and Delayed Union: Surgical Techniques

cortical screw because it was specifically designed for fixation of scaphoid fractures and can be accurately inserted using special instrumentation.[4] Furthermore, the screw can be inserted directly through the articular surface and buried within the bone so that it does not need to be removed later. This means that rigid fixation of small proximal pole fractures can be accomplished using the direct dorsal approach. Although adequate compression and fixation can be achieved with freehand insertion of the screw, the use of the jig is normally recommended.

The jig clamps around the scaphoid, holding the two fragments reduced and compressed during drilling, tapping, and insertion of the screw (Figure 6-5). When correctly applied, this instrument ensures that the screw is accurately positioned within the bone, and the instrument is calibrated to give a direct indication of the length of screw required. The jig is designed for use through the volar approach; it cannot be used when fixing small proximal pole fractures using the dorsal approach.

It takes some skill to learn how to apply the jig accurately, so that the screw is correctly placed perpendicular to the fracture and into the apex of the proximal pole. Practise with the jig on cadaver wrists is strongly recommended; even when one is familiar with the instrument's

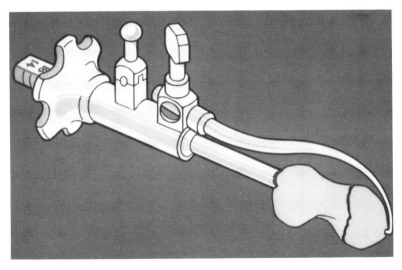

Figure 6-5. Jig used to hold the two fragments of the scaphoid firmly reduced during instrumentation and insertion of the Herbert screw.

use, certain fractures are so oblique or unstable that freehand insertion of the screw is more suitable.

To apply the jig, adequately mobilise the scaphotrapezial joint as previously described. Once the fracture has been reduced and stabilised, carefully pass the tip of the blade between the radius and the scaphoid and direct the blade towards the back of the wrist. Firm distraction on the hand opens up the radiocarpal joint, allowing a good view of the proximal pole of the scaphoid and ensuring that the tip of the blade can be positioned accurately. Position the hook of the blade on the *dorsal aspect* of the proximal pole, just to the radial side of the scapholunate joint. Engage the hook and hold it in position by applying gentle traction to the instrument whilst releasing traction on the wrist. The blade should lie snugly around the radial border of the scaphoid without impinging on the radius.

Elevate the distal pole of the scaphoid slightly, if necessary, using a small instrument designed for this purpose. Lock the guide of the jig onto the distal part of the bone by applying firm thumb pressure. If alignment of the guide appears satisfactory and the fracture remains anatomically reduced, obtain further compression by pushing firmly on

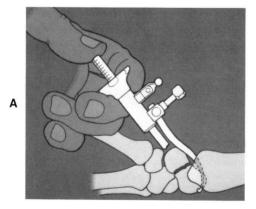
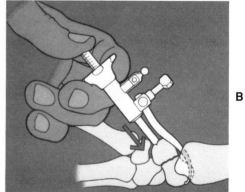

Figure 6-6. Application of the jig. **A,** The hook of the blade is engaged on the *dorsal* aspect of the proximal pole. **B,** The fracture is compressed by pressure applied to the guide of the jig. Note that the jig lies at an angle of at least 45 degrees to the long axis of the limb.

the drill guide. When seen from the side, the jig should lie at an angle of at least 45 degrees to the long axis of the limb (the normal angle of anteversion of the scaphoid) (Figure 6-6).

Again, carefully check the jig alignment to ensure that the screw will pass down the long axis of the scaphoid and will not penetrate medially or dorsally (Figure 6-7).

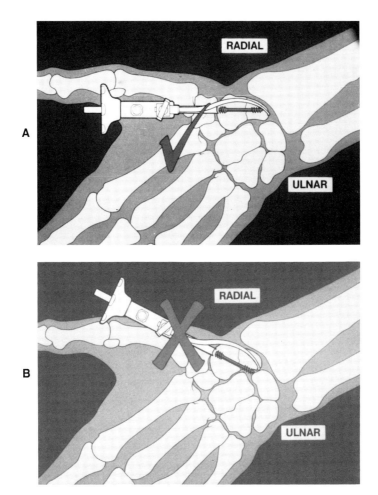

Figure 6-7. **A,** Jig applied in correct alignment so that the screw passes down the long axis of the scaphoid perpendicular to the fracture. **B,** The screw penetrates the scaphoid medially if the jig alignment is incorrect.

Chapter 6

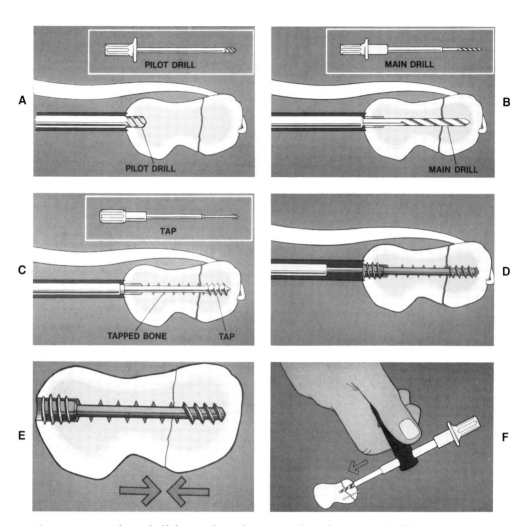

Figure 6-8. A, Short drill for trailing the screw thread. **B,** Long drill for leading the screw thread. **C,** Tap for leading the screw thread. **D,** Screw inserted through the jig. **E,** After removal of the jig, extra compression is achieved by tightening the screw another two turns. **F,** Method of freehand insertion of the Herbert screw using manual compression on the drill guide. In this case, a proximal pole fracture is being fixed using a dorsal approach. Note the temporary Kirschner wire to stabilise the fracture whilst the screw is being inserted.

Drill and tap the bone by hand in the recommended manner (Figure 6-8, *A* to *E*); select a screw of appropriate length and insert it through the jig. If the jig was incorrectly applied, penetration of the bone during drilling and tapping is indicated by loss of the normal resistance. If this occurs, remove the jig and insert the screw by the freehand method (Figure 6-8, *F*). Assuming satisfactory positioning of the screw, increase the compression by tightening the screw another one or two turns after removal of the jig, which ensures that the head is deeply buried. At this stage the fracture should be rigidly fixed. Smooth over the entry hole of the screw and check the fixation by manipulating the wrist.

Whatever method of internal fixation has been used, it is advisable to check the positioning of the implant and reduction of the fracture using either intraoperative x-ray studies or the image intensifier (Figure 6-9).

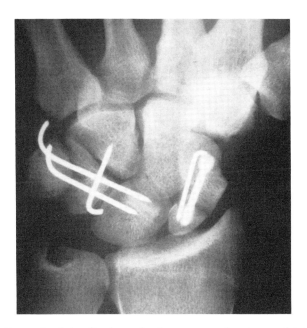

Figure 6-9. Radiograph of the final result after open reduction and internal fixation for a complex fracture dislocation of the wrist. Note the supplementary Kirschner wire fixation in the scaphoid and the use of additional Kirschner wires to stabilise the triquetrohamate and triquetrolunate joints after capsular repair.

Soft Tissue Repair and Wound Closure

The wrist capsule and volar radiocarpal ligaments must be carefully sutured using a fine (4-0) nonabsorbable suture. A fracture dislocation normally produces an extensive transverse tear across the volar wrist capsule, which requires careful repair. At this stage the carpal stability should be assessed. I have not normally found it necessary to repair the dorsal capsule as well, unless a combined approach to the wrist has been used. However, the integrity of the triquetrolunate and triquetrohamate joints should be tested, and, if necessary, these joints should be stabilised by capsular repair and temporary Kirschner wire fixation (see Figure 6-9).

Since the aim of surgery is to avoid postoperative joint immobilisation, the soft tissue repair should be sufficiently strong to allow the joint to be moved without the risk of creating instability. I have found that this always can be achieved by means of a meticulous suturing technique using nonabsorbable sutures that are strong enough to allow early joint mobilisation. I have never seen evidence of repair failure during the healing period.

POSTOPERATIVE MANAGEMENT

Assuming that satisfactory fixation has been achieved, joint motion should be started as soon as possible. Early joint motion encourages healing of damaged articular cartilage and prevents formation of intra-articular adhesions, leading to joint stiffness. Postoperative immobilisation in a plaster cast should be avoided.

Apply a firm bandage and use a volar slab to hold the wrist in the functional position (20 to 30 degrees of extension). Elevate the limb and start active finger exercises immediately. In the case of a relatively straightforward fracture with minimal intra-articular damage, the bandage may be left in place until the wound is healed, at 10 to 12 days, when active wrist exercises are commenced. With severe fractures, particularly those with significant intra-articular damage, considerable benefits accrue from starting joint motion after 48 hours. If the patient has difficulty moving the joint, a continuous passive motion device may be

Acute Fractures and Delayed Union: Surgical Techniques

useful. A volar resting splint may be used between exercise periods, but this should be removed at regular intervals (Figure 6-10, *A*). In the case of a fracture dislocation, I recommend the use of a limited motion wrist splint. This can be adjusted to allow some joint motion without stressing the repaired ligament (Figure 6-10, *B*).

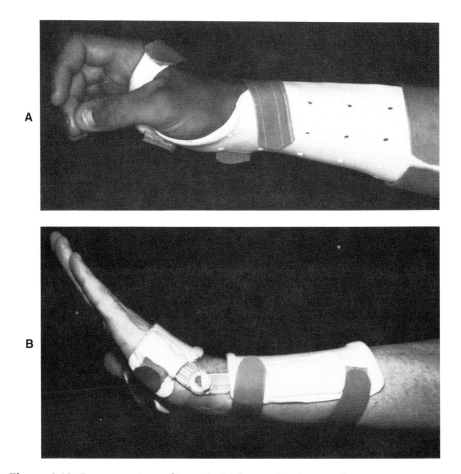

Figure 6-10. Postoperative splints. **A,** Lightweight thermoplastic removable splint used to protect the scaphoid from overloading during the healing period. The splint is removed for joint exercises. **B,** Hinged, limited-motion wrist splint used to protect soft tissue repair whilst allowing some joint motion following surgery for fracture dislocations. (Courtesy R. Prosser, B.Ap.Sc.Phy.)

Chapter 6

The fracture should not be overstressed during the first 6 weeks after surgery, by which time x-ray examination should confirm that bone union is proceeding satisfactorily (Figure 6-11). Patients may resume normal clerical work and even swimming as soon as the wound has healed. However, hard labour, the use of hammers and power tools, and contact sports must be avoided until there is evidence of bone healing. If there is a risk that the wrist may be overloaded within the first 6 weeks, the patient is advised to wear a suitable removable support. Patients are referred for physical therapy only if signs of joint stiffness or other problems develop. A hand therapist is the best person to assess the patient's fitness for return to work and to provide the most appropriate splint.

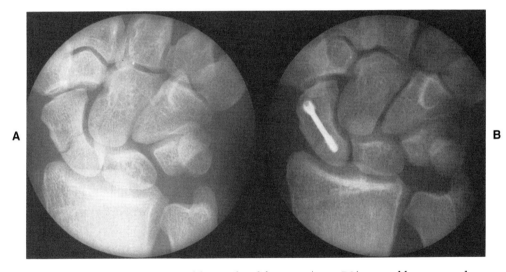

Figure 6-11. A, An acute unstable scaphoid fracture (type B2) treated by open reduction and internal fixation. **B,** X-ray at 6 weeks after surgery, showing advanced bone union.

Follow-up x-ray films are taken again at 12 weeks, by which time the fracture should be soundly united. At this stage the patient may resume full normal activities (Figure 6-12).

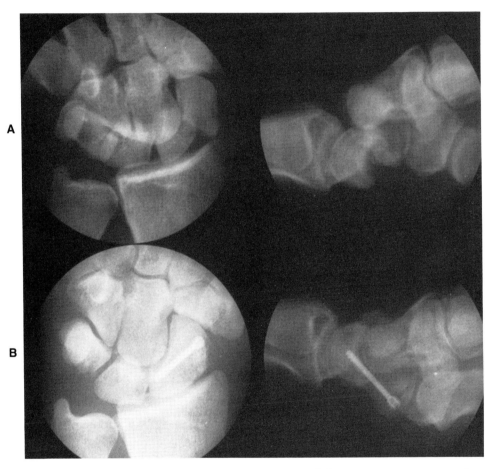

Figure 6-12. Results of open reduction and internal fixation in a patient with a transscaphoid-perilunate fracture dislocation of the carpus (**A**). An x-ray film 12 weeks after surgery (**B**) shows sound union of the fracture and normal alignment of the carpus. This patient regained normal function and a full range of motion in the wrist.

Chapter 6

RESULTS AND COMPLICATIONS

Provided that the operation has been carried out correctly, complications are few. Care should be taken to avoid damage to the palmar cutaneous branch of the median nerve when using the anterior approach and to the cutaneous branches of the radial nerve when using the lateral or dorsal approach. I have seen only one case of reflex sympathetic dystrophy after internal fixation of the scaphoid, and this appeared to be triggered by an ill-placed suture around the palmar cutaneous nerve. The wound was reexplored and the suture removed a few weeks later, after which the problem resolved quite rapidly.

In a series of 60 acute fractures and fracture dislocations treated by primary internal fixation, I have had two nonunions. In both cases, satisfactory reduction and fixation were achieved at the time of surgery, and failure was associated with late onset of avascular necrosis (Figure 6-13). This diagnosis did not become apparent for many months and in both cases the proximal fragment ultimately had to be replaced.

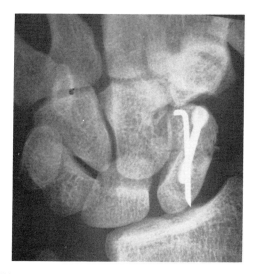

Figure 6-13. X-ray films to show developing nonunion 6 months after internal fixation of an acute unstable scaphoid fracture (type B1). Note change in bone density and loss of normal trabecular pattern, suggestive of impending avascular necrosis. A halo appearance around the leading screw thread indicates loss of fixation due to bone resorption.

In one patient a VISI instability pattern persisted after open reduction and internal fixation of a volar fracture dislocation, presumably because of inadequate repair of the ulnar carpal ligaments. Viegas[5] reported a similar problem in his series. Another patient required triquetrohamate fusion for persistent ulnar carpal instability after a severe fracture dislocation.

In many cases, the proximal fragment may appear relatively dense on x-ray studies for several months after injury, but this does not appear to affect healing, and the radiographical appearance of the scaphoid eventually returns to normal. I believe that the appearance of density of the proximal pole of the scaphoid, whilst indicating some degree of ischaemia of the bone, does not mean that it has undergone complete avascular necrosis (Figure 6-14). Comparison with x-ray studies of the

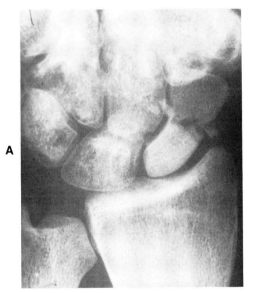
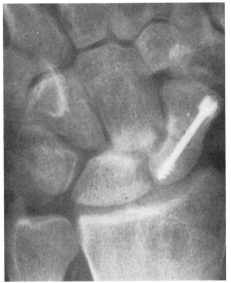

Figure 6-14. A, Radiograph after 8 weeks of immobilisation in a plaster cast for an acute unstable fracture of the scaphoid (type B2). The proximal fragment appears dense in relation to the surrounding osteoporosis, indicating a degree of ischaemia. **B,** After bone grafting and screw fixation, the fracture has united and the bone has regained a normal appearance. (From Herbert TJ, Fisher WE. Management of the fractured scaphoid using a new bone screw. J Bone Joint Surg 66B:114, 1984.)

opposite wrist show that this density is, in fact, normal, whereas other bones in the wrist have become osteoporotic as a result of disuse. When true avascular necrosis occurs, the proximal fragment appears cystic and deformed on x-ray examination (see Chapter 8).

A close analogy may be drawn between scaphoid fractures and subcapital fractures of the femoral neck. These injuries always carry a risk of avascular necrosis, particularly if the trauma has been severe or if anatomical variances result in an unusually precarious blood supply to the proximal fragment. Although open reduction and internal fixation cannot be guaranteed to prevent this complication, most would agree that surgery is the best way of reducing this risk.

After closed treatment of fracture dislocations, avascular necrosis of the scaphoid is almost inevitable. To date it has not occurred in any of those cases that have been treated surgically.

REFERENCES

1. Russe, O. Fracture of the carpal navicular: Diagnosis, nonoperative treatment and operative treatment. J Bone Joint Surg 42A:759, 1960.
2. Fisk, E. Carpal instability in the fractured scaphoid. Ann R Coll Surg Engl 46:63, 1970.
3. Bohler J, Ender HG. Die pseudoarthrose des scaphoid. Orthopaede 15:109, 1986.
4. Herbert TJ. Surgical Technique. The Herbert Bone Screw, rev. ed. Warsaw, Ind.: Zimmer, Inc., Technical Publication, 1987.
5. Viegas SF, Hoffman FJ. Palmar lunate dislocation with a dorsal scaphoid fracture variant. J Hand Surg 13A:440, 1988.

7

Treatment of Established Nonunion

The decision whether or not to operate on
a scaphoid pseudarthrosis depends on a number
of factors, including the patient's age, the
degree of disability, and the extent of the
deformity and secondary arthritis.

It is important to differentiate between a stable and an unstable scaphoid nonunion (see Classification of Scaphoid Fractures, Chapter 5). *The stable scaphoid nonunion* (type D1) is characterised by a firm fibrous union that prevents deformity from occurring. The length and shape of the scaphoid remain well preserved and the risk of osteoarthritis is minimal. X-ray studies normally show an indistinct fracture line with variable cystic changes affecting the adjacent bone fragments (Figure 7-1). The patient may be relatively, but rarely completely, symptom free unless the wrist is subjected to further trauma, which then may lead to the development of an unstable pseudarthrosis. At surgery these fractures are often remarkably stable and indeed the articular cartilage may appear to have healed. However, synovial adhesions should lead to the fracture site. I suspect that tension on these adhesions is the most likely explanation of the discomfort these patients experience on stressing the wrist.

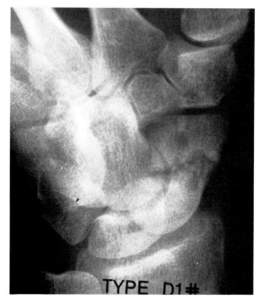

Figure 7-1. X-ray appearance of a stable fibrous union (type D1). Note the cystic change adjacent to the fracture and the absence of significant deformity. (From Herbert TJ. Use of the Herbert bone screw in surgery of the wrist. Clin Orthop 202:79, 1986.)

In contrast, an *unstable scaphoid nonunion,* or pseudarthrosis (Type D2), is nearly always associated with some degree of carpal collapse deformity and secondary osteoarthritis. Depending on the age of the fracture, the bone faces tend to become sclerotic, with synovial erosion and fibrous cysts extending into both bone fragments. As the fracture surfaces abrade each other, a deformity develops, leading to a marked discrepancy between the diameter of the two bone fragments (Figure 7-2). In extreme cases, only a small fragment of proximal bone remains, even though the original fracture may have been through the waist of the scaphoid.

The prognosis following surgery in type D1 fractures is excellent, whereas in type D2 fractures the result depends on the viability of the bone fragments and the extent to which secondary changes have developed.

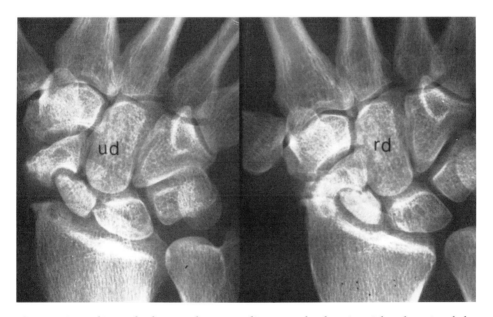

Figure 7-2. Radiograph shows a long-standing pseudarthrosis with sclerosis of the fracture faces (type D2). There is marked deformity with discrepancy in the size of the two fragments. The osteophyte formation on the distal fragment is associated with radiocarpal osteoarthritis. Note instability of fracture demonstrated on ulnar (*ud*) and radial (*rd*) deviation of the wrist.

Chapter 7

Staging the nonunion according to its radiological appearance assists the surgeon in determining the prognosis and deciding whether reconstructive surgery is indicated (see chart below).

Reconstruction is indicated in *stage 1*, even if the patient is asymptomatic, since successful surgery prevents further deterioration and improves the long-term prognosis.

In *stage 2*, reconstruction is normally indicated, unless the patient is over 50 years old and has only minimal symptoms.

Staging of Scaphoid Nonunions

	Stage 1	Stage 2
Type	Fibrous union (D1)	Pseudarthrosis (D2)
X-ray appearance		
Fracture mobility	±	+
Loss of bone stock	0	+
Carpal collapse deformity	0	+
Loss of motion	±	+
Osteoarthritis	0	+
Union rate	++++	+++

Note: All cases of previous failed surgery should be classified one stage worse than that suggested by x-ray appearance.

Patients with *stage 3* pseudarthrosis should undergo reconstruction only if their symptoms are severe enough to impair function.

In *stages 4 and 5,* reconstruction is normally contraindicated and the choice of procedure depends on the patient's symptoms (see Chapters 8 and 9).

In all cases where previous surgery has failed, bone stock is usually poor even if no osteoarthritis and minimal deformity are present. These cases should be classified as one stage worse than that suggested by the radiological appearance when deciding whether further reconstruction is justified.

Stage 3	Stage 4	Stage 5
Pseudarthrosis	Pseudarthrosis	Avascular necrosis
++	+++	*
++	+++	++++
++	+++	*
++	+++	++++
++	+++	*
++	+	0

*Depends on age of fracture and amount of previous treatment, if any.

TREATMENT OF FIBROUS UNION (TYPE D1)
Indications

Even if the patient is asymptomatic, I believe that all fibrous unions should be treated by bone grafting.

If left untreated, the fibrous union is likely to become unstable over time, leading to the development of pseudarthrosis and secondary osteoarthritis. The prognosis should be explained carefully so that the patient understands the need to undergo reconstructive surgery before the wrist starts to deteriorate.

Surgical Technique
Incision

For distal oblique and waist fractures the volar approach is preferred (see Chapter 6). For small proximal fractures the dorsal approach provides better access.

Fracture Preparation

Free synovial adhesions from the fracture site, which is then gently prised open using a sharp dissector (Figure 7-3). If the articular cartilage has healed and the fracture site is not immediately apparent, obtain intraoperative x-ray films to avoid unnecessary damage when locating the fracture.

Remove all fibrous tissue and unhealthy looking bone using small rongeurs and a fine, angled curette. Sometimes the cysts extend a long way into both bone fragments; it is important to thoroughly clear the cysts so that healthy cancellous bone appears on both fracture faces. In the case of small proximal pole fractures, take care not to remove too much bone from the proximal fragment since this may jeopardise fixation.

Treatment of Established Nonunion

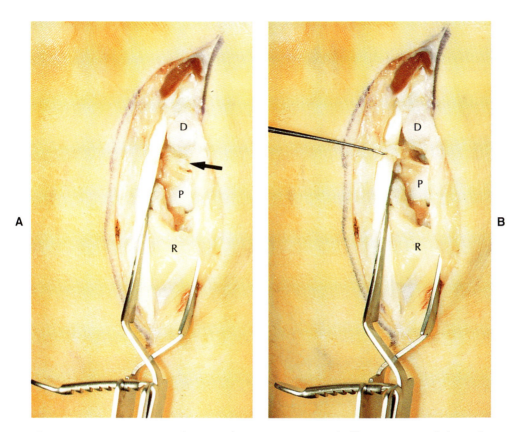

Figure 7-3. Intraoperative photographs in a patient with fibrous union of the right scaphoid. **A,** The scaphoid is exposed through the standard volar approach (*D*, distal pole; *P,* proximal pole; *R,* radius). Note the synovial adhesions at the fracture site (arrow). **B,** The fracture has been prised open and a fold of synovium is being lifted out from between the bone fragments.

Chapter 7

Bone Grafting

Use a fresh cancellous bone graft to pack any defects in the proximal and distal fragments. If a significant amount of bone was removed from the fracture itself, use a small corticocancellous block to maintain normal length of the scaphoid and prevent malunion. If the articular surfaces can be closely apposed without deformity, then an

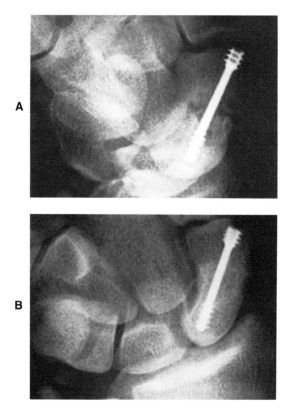

Figure 7-4. A, Radiographical appearance approximately 6 months after internal fixation of a fibrous union in which no bone graft was used. Note the signs of persistent nonunion with cystic changes adjacent to the fracture and screw loosening. B, Radiograph after reconstructive surgery that involved removal of the implant, curettage of the fracture, cancellous bone grafting, and rigid internal fixation. This fracture went on to rapid union without plaster immobilisation.

interposition graft is unnecessary, although sufficient cancellous bone must be packed into the fracture to eliminate residual spaces. I normally recommend the use of an iliac crest bone graft because its osteogenic and mechanical properties are infinitely superior to those of the distal radius or proximal ulna. Occasionally, when exploring a fibrous union, the fracture appears to be soundly healed. However, if the x-ray films show any degree of cystic change at the fracture site, the surgeon must prise open the fibrous union and curette and graft the fracture in the normal way. Internal fixation alone cannot compress the fracture because of the intact articular cartilage, and nonunion almost certainly will persist unless the fracture is grafted (Figure 7-4).

Fixation

After grafting and accurate reduction of the scaphoid, carry out internal fixation using whatever method is preferred (Chapter 6). Although early joint motion is not as important as it is after treatment of acute fractures, it is preferable to avoid postoperative plaster immobilisation if possible. The patient with an asymptomatic nonunion will particularly appreciate being allowed to use the wrist again as soon as the wound has healed. Thus compression fixation appears to be the best method of immobilising the scaphoid during the healing period. When using the Herbert bone screw system, application of the jig is relatively simple, and excellent compression can normally be achieved.

Postoperative Management

The postoperative management depends on the method of fixation used, but early joint mobilisation prevents intra-articular adhesions and joint stiffness and appears to accelerate union.

Results

X-ray films taken 6 weeks after surgery normally show good incorporation of the bone graft with early bone union, which should be complete within 12 weeks (Figure 7-5). Provided that no carpal collapse occurred preoperatively, the patient can expect to regain a full range of motion and normal wrist function.

Chapter 7

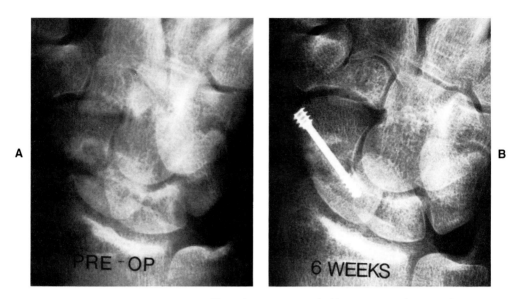

Figure 7-5. A, Preoperative x-ray film of a patient with fibrous union (type D1). **B,** Six weeks after bone grafting and compression screw fixation, the x-ray film showed good incorporation of the graft. By this time the patient had regained almost normal function of the wrist.

TREATMENT OF SCAPHOID PSEUDARTHROSIS (TYPE D2)
Indications

The decision whether or not to operate on a scaphoid pseudarthrosis depends on a number of factors, including the patient's age, the degree of disability, and the extent of the deformity and secondary arthritis. Reconstruction is normally indicated in stages 2 and 3 (see pp. 94-95).

Principles of Reconstructive Surgery

It is useful to define the aims of treatment:
1. *To correct the carpal collapse deformity* as completely as possible. This should improve the range of motion and reduce the risk of osteoarthritis.

2. *To stabilise the carpus* by internal fixation of the scaphoid reinforced by obtaining sound bony union.
3. *To relieve symptoms* arising as a result of localised osteoarthritis.

Thus reconstructive surgery involves complete resection of the pseudarthrosis, correction of the carpal collapse deformity, and restoration of length to the scaphoid using an adequate corticocancellous bone graft. Good internal fixation maintains the correction and enhances healing. Arthritic joint surfaces should be unloaded or decompressed when possible.

In the case of proximal pole pseudarthrosis, it may not be possible to apply all of these principles. Fortunately, carpal collapse and secondary osteoarthritis are relatively rare with this type of fracture, although nonunion is the rule. It is not feasible to use an interpositional bone graft when the proximal fragment is extremely small. Under these circumstances, I prefer to stabilise the fracture by screw fixation from the dorsal approach, with or without cancellous bone grafting, depending on the findings at the time of surgery. Even though many of these fractures are unlikely to unite, the sclerotic bone allows for good internal fixation, and stabilisation of the fracture usually relieves most of the patient's symptoms. I agree with Green[1] that the number of punctate bleeding points is a good indicator of vascularity of the bone, and it is not until this stage that the surgeon can make an accurate prognosis for bone healing. Even if the bone appears completely sclerotic (ischaemic), I always proceed with scaphoid reconstruction, provided the bone stock in the proximal fragment is adequate for good internal fixation. Although the fracture may not unite, the patient's own bone is better than any implant. Against all expectations, some of these cases do achieve sound bony union (Figure 7-6). Nothing is lost by adopting a "wait-and-see" policy, since revision surgery can always be carried out later. In many ways, reattachment of the ischaemic proximal fragment resembles the technique of scaphoid allografting recently reported by Carter et al.[2] Reattachment of the fragment has all of the advantages and none of the disadvantages of allografts. Although this approach does nothing for one's "union rate," I firmly believe that it is in the patient's best interests.

Chapter 7

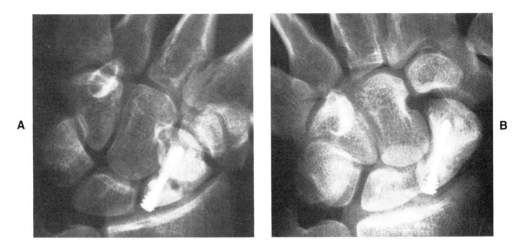

Figure 7-6. A, X-ray appearance of the scaphoid 1 year after cancellous bone grafting and retrograde screw fixation for long-standing pseudarthrosis of a proximal pole fracture (stage 4). No evidence of union exists, but the screw appears to be maintaining satisfactory fixation. The patient was asymptomatic and resumed playing professional sport. **B,** X-ray appearance 1 year later. Although the views are not strictly comparable, union appears to have occurred despite a halo around the proximal screw thread. The patient has remained asymptomatic and the screw has not been removed.

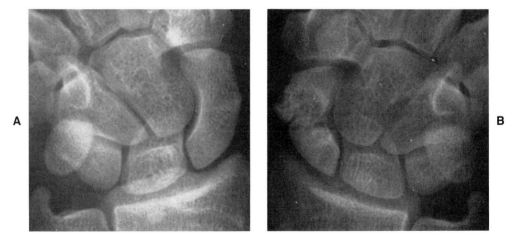

Figure 7-7. Preoperative x-rays of both wrists (**A,** left; **B,** right) show deformity and shortening of the right scaphoid resulting from an ununited fracture (type D2). The aim of surgery is to reconstruct the scaphoid using sufficient bone graft to restore normal length.

SCAPHOID RECONSTRUCTION
Surgical Technique

Careful preoperative planning is required to determine the degree of correction that one may expect to achieve. X-ray films documenting the amount of deformity and shortening of the scaphoid should be compared with films of the opposite normal wrist (Figure 7-7).

General anaesthesia is preferred, and the patient should be positioned with a sandbag under the opposite hip and the iliac crest prepared as the donor site for bone grafting.

Incision

The standard volar approach should be used for all reconstructions except those involving small proximal pole fractures (Chapter 6).

Fracture Preparation (Volar Approach)

Once the scaphoid has been exposed, free all adhesions and mobilise the fracture completely (Figure 7-8, *A*). Forcibly extend the wrist. This manoeuvre, combined with the use of small spreaders to open out the fracture, normally achieves an adequate correction of the carpal deformity and a satisfactory improvement in wrist extension. The limiting factor is the degree of volar capsular contracture and tethering of the lunate. I do not believe that any attempt should be made to release this contracture, since such a procedure could produce significant instability and may jeopardise the blood supply to the bone. Provided that reasonable correction is achieved and that the wrist extends to at least 45 degrees, most patients achieve satisfactory clinical results. However, I accept the fact that the risk of midcarpal arthritis developing remains unless the deformity has been corrected completely.

Use a small osteotome to excise the fracture faces (Figure 7-8, *B-C*). It is important that the cuts be parallel to each other and perpendicular to the long axis of the scaphoid to ensure that the graft is stable when it is locked into position. Whenever possible, preserve a shelf of bone or a soft tissue hinge posteriorly, since this shelf provides a fulcrum around which the fragments may be hinged open and considerably enhances the stability of the graft (Figure 7-8, *D*). Do not attempt removal of the dorsal osteophyte at this stage. Curette thoroughly any remaining cysts or cavities in the body of the bone.

After the osteotomy, reassess and note the viability of the bone fragments. In most waist fractures the bone surfaces should appear reasonably healthy once the pseudarthrosis has been excised. However, the smaller the proximal fragment, the more likely it is that the body of the bone will be sclerotic.

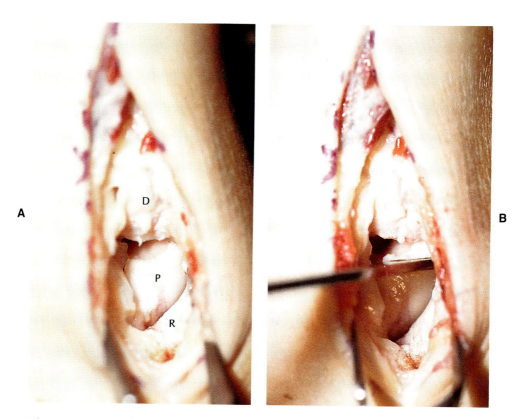

Figure 7-8. Surgical technique for reconstruction of a scaphoid pseudarthrosis using a volar approach, right wrist. **A,** The scaphoid has been exposed through the standard volar approach and the capsule has been retracted to show the pseudarthrosis. *D,* Distal fragment; *P,* proximal fragment; *R,* radius. **B,** Osteotomy of the sclerotic proximal fracture face.

Bone Graft

Take the bone graft from the opposite iliac crest. I infiltrate the area with 0.5% bupivacaine (Marcaine) and epinephrine because these drugs help reduce bleeding and relieve much of the postoperative pain associated with this procedure. Make a 6 to 8 cm skin incision along the lateral border of the iliac crest, starting a short distance behind the anterior superior iliac spine. Divide the deep fascia and detach the muscles from the outer aspect of the iliac crest. Make a transverse osteotomy across the apex of the crest, again staying a few centimetres behind the

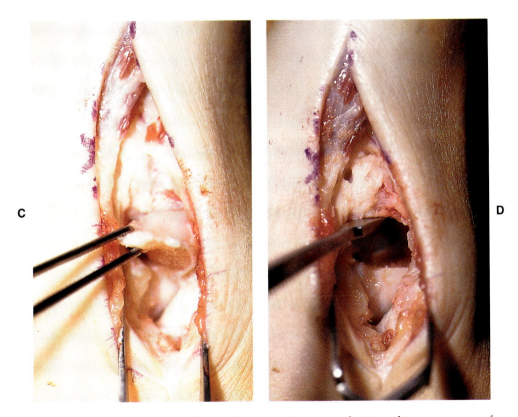

Figure 7-8, cont'd. C, The sclerotic fragment is removed. Note the appearance of viable cancellous bone in the proximal pole. **D,** The fracture faces have been excised and a soft tissue hinge has been preserved posteriorly. Note the size of the defect when the wrist is fully extended to correct the deformity. *Continued.*

Chapter 7

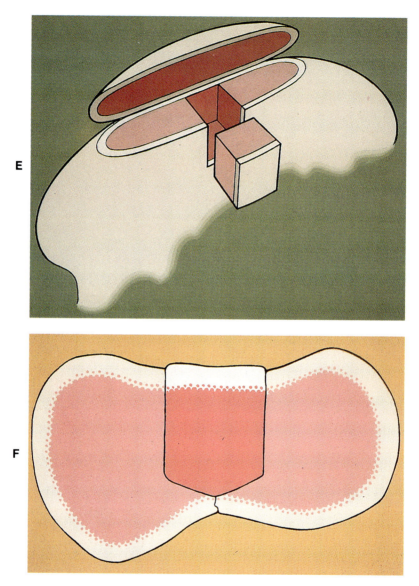

Figure 7-8, cont'd. E, Technique for obtaining a suitable corticocancellous bone block from the iliac crest. **F,** The graft should be fashioned to fit accurately into the defect. Note how the cortex of the graft lies flush with the volar cortex of the scaphoid.

Treatment of Established Nonunion

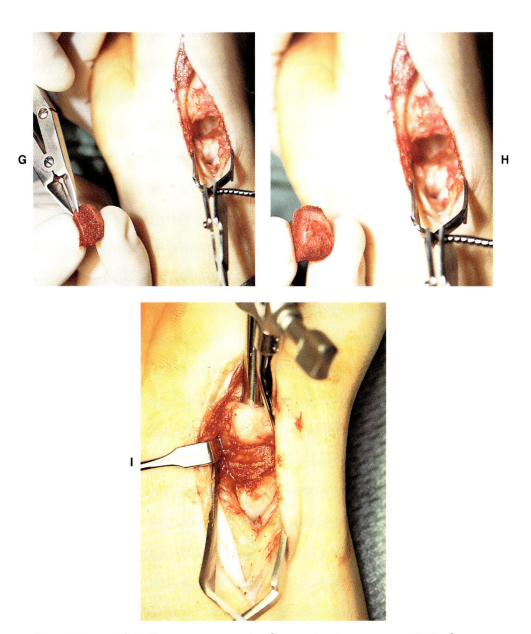

Figure 7-8, cont'd. G, Bone carpentry using fine cutting instruments. **H,** Final assessment of the graft before insertion into the scaphoid. Note that the wrist is held in full extension to maintain correction of the deformity. **I,** After application of the jig, the scaphoid has been compressed. The graft is firmly locked into position.

Continued.

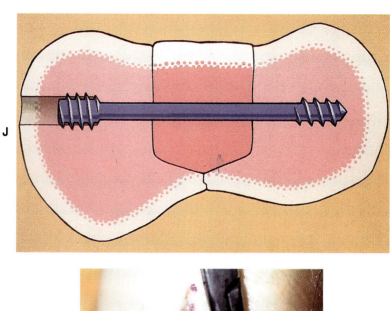

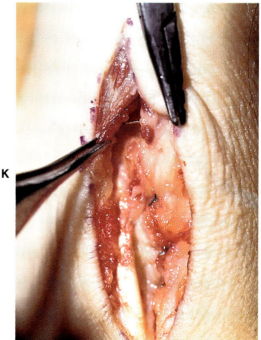

Figure 7-8, cont'd. J, The bone graft is compressed and locked into position once the screw has been inserted and fully tightened. **K,** Closure of the capsule and volar radiocarpal ligaments has been carried out using fine (4-0) nonabsorbable sutures.

anterior superior iliac spine to avoid damage to the lateral cutaneous nerve of the thigh. Use a broad osteotome to lever up the crest and gently tap it down the inner border for a few centimetres so that it acts as a retractor. It is then possible to cut a suitable block of corticocancellous bone from the outer table of the ilium using small osteotomes (Figure 7-8, *E*). Cut the block larger than the size of the graft required, bearing in mind that the outer cortex forms the new volar surface of the scaphoid. Leave the inner table of the iliac crest intact, provided that the depth of the graft is adequate to fill the scaphoid defect. Carefully remove the bone block and store it in a small bowl containing the patient's blood to maintain the bone's viability. At this stage, a curette may be used to obtain further cancellous graft should additional bone be needed to fill defects or cavities in the proximal and distal fragments of the scaphoid. Secure haemostasis by applying bone wax on the raw bone surface; reposition and reattach the hinged "lid" of the iliac crest using strong sutures between the periosteum and deep fascia overlying the muscles. A suction drain prevents haematoma formation.

Using fine rongeurs and bone cutters, carefully shape the bone graft to fit into the defect created in the scaphoid when the wrist is in maximal extension (Figure 7-8, *G-H*). The proximal and distal faces of the graft should be flat, to fit snugly against the two fracture faces, and the borders rounded so they do not protrude outside the bone. Adjust the graft depth to make the cortical surface flush with the volar cortex of the scaphoid (Figure 7-8, *F*).

It is extremely important that this bone carpentry is carried out accurately. A snug graft fit holds the scaphoid in its corrected, elongated position. Normally a small punch is used to impact the graft, at which stage the bone should be quite stable. Again check extension of the wrist and palpate the scaphoid with a curved dissector to ensure that the graft does not protrude beyond the bone.

Internal Fixation

Again, the method of internal fixation depends on the choice of the surgeon. The simplest method is to use two Kirschner wires; however, these do not provide compression so union is likely to be slow. Rigid internal fixation is preferable. With the Herbert Bone Screw System, the jig can produce extremely strong compression, which locks the

Chapter 7

graft firmly in position and prevents movement at the graft-fracture interfaces (Figure 7-8, *I*). When the screw has been fully inserted, further compression is achieved and fixation should be absolutely rigid (Figures 7-8, *J*, and 7-9). However, if the graft tends to rotate, provide additional fixation with a single Kirschner wire. Both the screw and the wire should cross the graft and obtain a firm hold in the proximal fragment (Figure 7-10).

At the end of the procedure, check fixation again and carefully trim prominent bone graft so that the surface of the scaphoid is completely smooth. Note the degree of wrist extension achieved and take intraoperative x-ray films at this stage to confirm the implant position and show the degree of correction achieved (Figure 7-11). No gap should be visible at either fracture interface.

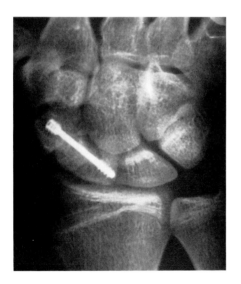

Figure 7-9

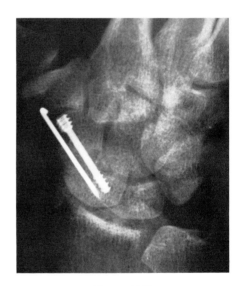

Figure 7-10

Figure 7-9. X-ray film taken immediately after scaphoid reconstruction using an interpositional bone graft and compression screw fixation. Note the graft size and the degree of compression achieved so that both interfaces are closely apposed.

Figure 7-10. X-ray film shows the use of a supplementary Kirschner wire to enhance stability of the bone graft after scaphoid reconstruction.

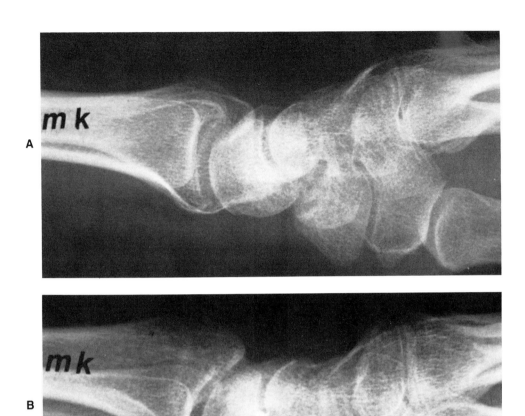

Figure 7-11. A, Preoperative x-ray appearance of a patient with a 2-year-old unstable scaphoid nonunion (stage 3). Note the associated carpal collapse deformity with dorsiflexed lunate (DISI pattern). B, X-ray appearance after scaphoid reconstruction. The cortical portion of the iliac crest graft is clearly seen. Carpal alignment is improved, and almost complete correction of the previous lunate dorsiflexion deformity has been accomplished. Wrist extension was improved from 40 to 80 degrees.

Chapter 7

Closure

Carefully close the wrist capsule and volar radiocarpal ligaments with fine nonabsorbable sutures (see Figure 7-8, *K*). Use a single horizontal mattress suture to reattach soft tissues to the tubercle distally; it is not necessary to attempt a separate repair of the scaphotrapezial joint capsule.

SMALL PROXIMAL POLE FRACTURES
Surgical Technique (Figure 7-12)

The direct dorsal approach is used to operate on small proximal pole fractures (Figure 7-12, *A*). After exposing the fracture (Figure 7-12, *B-C*), carefully curette out the pseudarthrosis. The proximal fragment never has enough bone to allow for an osteotomy. Curette any cysts extending into the distal fragment and pack all cavities with fresh cancellous bone graft. The graft should be sufficient to close the gap between the two fragments but no attempt should be made to lengthen the scaphoid. I look upon the proximal pole of the scaphoid as being an osteochondral fragment, which may be reattached by closely apposing the adjacent articular surfaces. Hold the fragment in position with a temporary Kirschner wire (Figure 7-12, *D*), and try to maintain compression of the fracture by applying manual pressure to the drill guide whilst the screw is being inserted (Figure 7-12, *E*). A 16 or 18 mm screw is usually long enough to cross the fracture. Once the screw has been buried beneath the articular surface of the proximal fragment, carefully smooth the entry hole over (Figure 7-12, *G*) and remove the Kirschner wire. Intraoperative x-ray films are taken to confirm satisfactory positioning of the screw (Figure 7-13). Because the bone in the proximal fragment is nearly always sclerotic, the screw tends to retain a strong hold in the bone, even if the fracture is slow to heal. Repair the dorsal wrist capsule with fine nonabsorbable sutures.

Text continued on p. 118.

Treatment of Established Nonunion

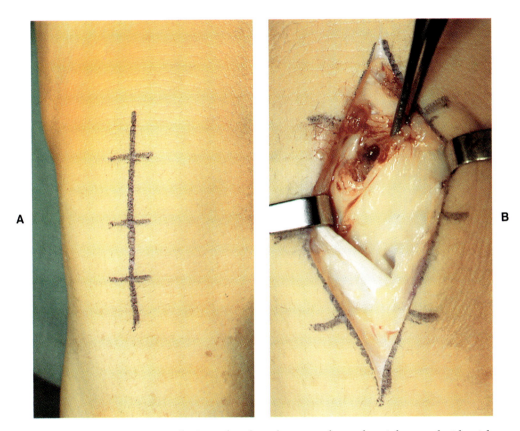

Figure 7-12. Operative technique for dorsal approach to the right scaphoid with freehand screw fixation for proximal pole fracture. **A,** Skin incision centred over proximal pole of scaphoid. **B,** Extensor pollicis longus tendon is retracted radially; capsule has been opened. Note haemarthrosis. *Continued.*

Chapter 7

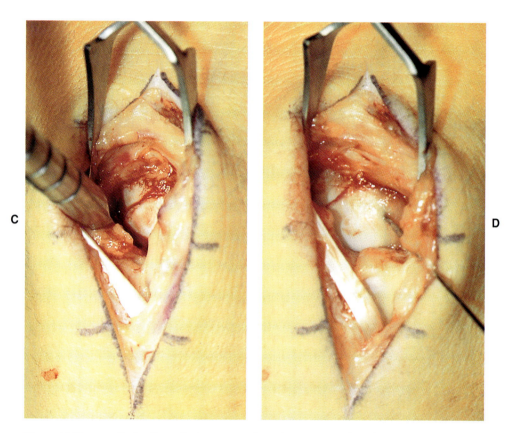

Figure 7-12, cont'd. C, Capsule is retracted to show a complete fracture through the proximal pole of the scaphoid. **D,** Fracture has been anatomically reduced and held with a Kirschner wire passed proximally to distally.

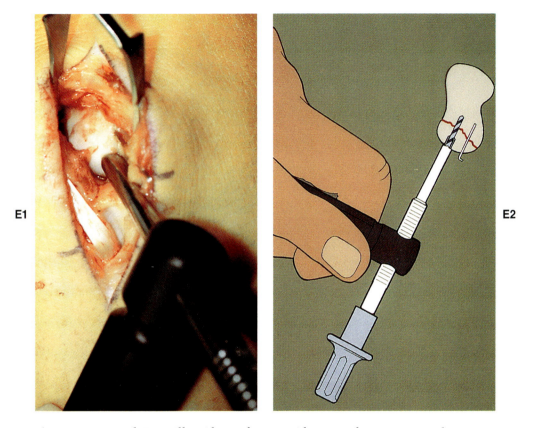

Figure 7-12, cont'd. E, Drill guide used to provide manual compression during instrumentation.

Continued.

Chapter 7

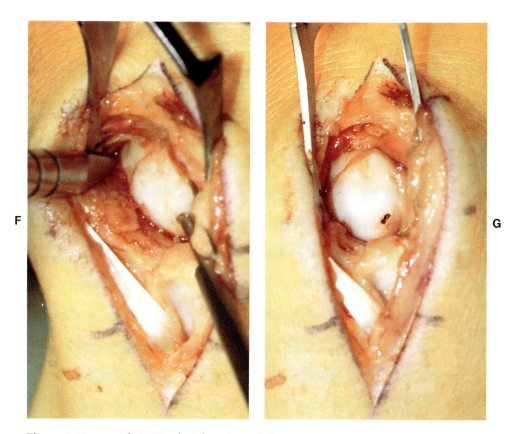

Figure 7-12, cont'd. F, Final tightening of the screw to increase compression. **G,** Appearance following screw fixation. Note compression at fracture and small defect in articular cartilage following insertion of screw. The temporary Kirschner wire has been removed.

Treatment of Established Nonunion

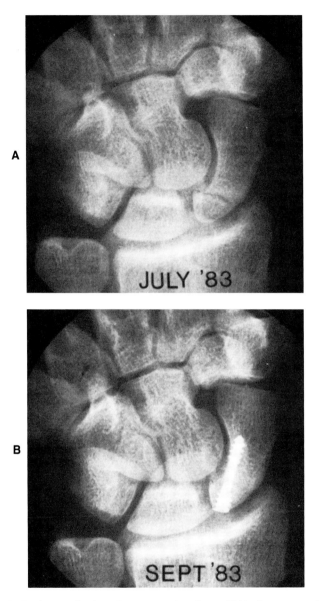

Figure 7-13. **A,** Radiograph showing nonunion (type D1) after a proximal pole fracture of the scaphoid. **B,** Appearance after cancellous bone grafting and compression screw fixation through a direct dorsal incision. The screw head is buried beneath the articular cartilage of the proximal fragment. (From Herbert TJ. Scaphoid fractures: Operative treatment. In Barton NJ, ed. Fractures of the Hand and Wrist. Edinburgh: Churchill Livingstone, 1988, p 225.)

Chapter 7

Postoperative Management

Provided that good internal fixation has been achieved, no postoperative immobilisation is required, and the patient is encouraged to start early mobilising exercises of the wrist. Most patients may return to work as soon as the wound has healed, but the repair should be protected from further trauma for at least 6 weeks. This means that the patient should not do heavy manual work, use power tools, play contact sports, or pursue hazardous occupations such as motorcycle racing and horse riding. Remarkably, in more than 300 cases of scaphoid reconstruction using this technique, I can recall only two instances in which postoperative trauma caused failure of union. One of these patients fell off his horse whilst riding in a rodeo a few days after surgery (against medical advice!). The second patient sustained a forceful twisting injury of the wrist whilst using a heavy power drill at work a few weeks after surgery.

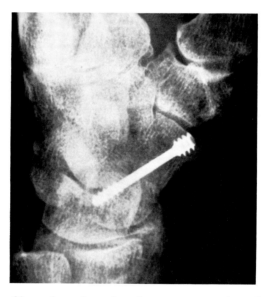

Figure 7-14. X-ray film taken 6 weeks after reconstruction of a scaphoid pseudarthrosis. No postoperative immobilisation was used. The graft appears well incorporated, and it is difficult to know whether union occurred. The patient made a full recovery with no sign of graft resorption.

I believe considerable benefits result from allowing patients to start using their wrists as soon as possible. The risk of intra-articular adhesions is minimised and the degree of wrist extension obtained at surgery is maintained. Disuse osteoporosis is avoided, which ensures that fixation remains secure. Furthermore, the bone graft appears to incorporate far more rapidly when the wrist is moved than when it is immobilised in a plaster cast. Indeed, in most cases it is hard to know when union has occurred, since there should be no gap at the graft-bone interfaces (Figure 7-14).

Check x-ray films are obtained at 6 and 12 weeks and thereafter as indicated; all patients are reviewed at 1 year. Graft resorption indicates failure of bone union (Figure 7-15). Eventually, some loosening of the screw is likely, although reasonable fixation may be maintained for many years, even if the fracture has not united. Nonunion nearly always occurs at the proximal interface, indicating that bone vascularity deter-

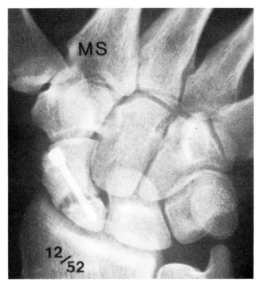

Figure 7-15. Radiograph showing bone graft resorption at 12 weeks after reconstructive surgery for a proximal pole pseudarthrosis. The proximal fragment appeared ischaemic at operation. Although this fracture failed to unite, the patient remains asymptomatic, presumably because the screw continues to provide adequate stability.

mines whether the fracture will heal. For this reason repeated grafting is pointless. If symptomatic nonunion persists in spite of adequate reconstruction, further surgery is directed towards relief of symptoms arising as a result of late avascular necrosis or secondary osteoarthrosis (see Chapter 9).

REFERENCES

1. Green, DP. The effect of avascular necrosis on Russe bone grafting for scaphoid non-union. J Hand Surg 10A:597-605, 1985.
2. Carter PR, Malinin TI, Abbey PA, Sommerkamp TG. The scaphoid allograft: A new operation for treatment of the very proximal scaphoid nonunion or for the necrotic, fragmented scaphoid proximal pole. J Hand Surg 14A:1, 1989.

8

Avascular Necrosis of the Scaphoid

When considering treatment, it is useful to compare avascular necrosis of the scaphoid with Kienböck's disease of the lunate.

Chapter 8

What is meant by the term "avascular necrosis"? Literally interpreted, it means "death of tissue due to cutting off its blood supply." Thus *avascular necrosis* of the scaphoid means complete (and therefore irreversible) death of the bone. That is, reconstruction is no longer possible. With tissue necrosis the dead bone is replaced by scar tissue, the normal trabecular structure disappears, and the bone tends to collapse and deform. At this stage, x-ray films show loss of trabeculation, cystic changes, and deformity of the bone (Figure 8-1).

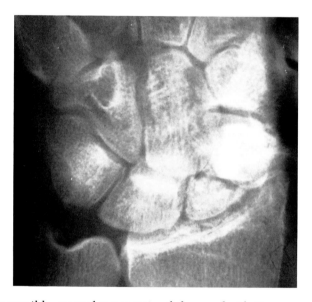

Figure 8-1. Irreversible avascular necrosis of the scaphoid. X-ray appearance of the scaphoid following failed bone graft for scaphoid nonunion. The associated carpal collapse deformity indicates a well-established pseudarthrosis. Note the loss of normal trabeculation, cystic change, and deformity of the small proximal fragment. At operation the bone was soft and not suitable for reconstruction.

This is in contrast to *ischaemic bone,* which appears dense on the x-ray film and sclerotic at the time of surgery (Figure 8-2). Dense bone is strong bone; it does not collapse under loading and can be stabilised by internal fixation. Healing, although likely to be slow, remains possible as long as a chance of revascularisation exists. I find it useful to think in terms of ischaemia changing the properties of medullary bone into those of cortical bone. It is therefore technically incorrect to use the term "avascular necrosis" to describe the radiological changes of increased bone density that commonly occur after a scaphoid fracture. These points have been emphasised by Carter et al.[1] in their excellent paper on scaphoid allografting.

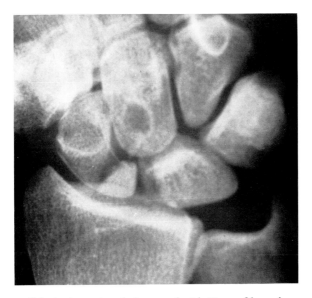

Figure 8-2. Reversible ischaemia of the scaphoid. X-ray film of an acute proximal pole fracture of the scaphoid (type B3) following immobilisation in a plaster cast for 3 months. Note the relative density of the proximal fragment in contrast with the surrounding osteoporosis. At surgery the proximal pole fragment was hard (ischaemic) and was suitable for internal fixation.

Chapter 8

DIAGNOSIS

Avascular necrosis occurs as a late complication of scaphoid fractures, especially those involving the proximal pole. It is particularly common when nonunion persists after unsuccessful bone grafting or poor internal fixation. Occasionally avascular necrosis may occur without a fracture, either as a complication of scapholunate ligament rupture or as an idiopathic condition in women called Preiser's disease (Figure 8-3).

The onset of avascular necrosis is heralded by increasing pain and stiffness of the wrist. Examination shows signs of an "irritable wrist joint" with tenderness and swelling over the back of the wrist due to chronic synovitis.

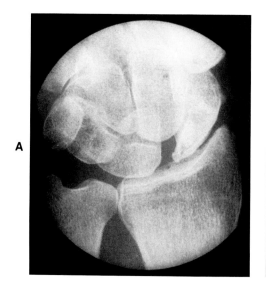
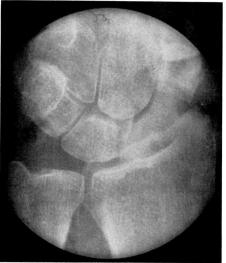

Figure 8-3. Preiser's disease. This patient had a history of increasing pain and stiffness in the wrist after nonspecific trauma. Examination showed an "irritable wrist" with acute synovitis. **A,** Radiograph shows typical appearance of avascular necrosis of the proximal half of the scaphoid (Preiser's disease) without fracture. Note, however, widening of the scapholunate joint due to attenuation of the scapholunate ligament. **B,** Appearance after prosthetic replacement of the proximal two thirds of the scaphoid (using a silicone implant).

X-ray examination normally shows a small, deformed proximal pole fragment. Cystic changes and areas of sclerosis are also likely, and loss of trabeculation may produce a "ground-glass" appearance (see Figure 8-1). Carpal collapse deformity and secondary degenerative changes are common, particularly in cases of well-established scaphoid pseudarthrosis.

Bone scans show intense uptake around the radiocarpal joint, and it is seldom possible to define the area of avascular bone. MRI, however, particularly in the early stages, may show a "black hole" (loss of normal fat shadow), which is said to be diagnostic of avascular necrosis (Figure 8-4).

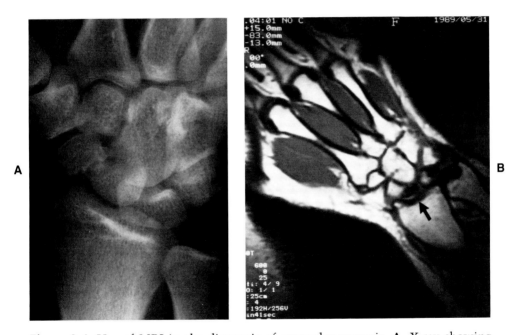

Figure 8-4. Use of MRI in the diagnosis of avascular necrosis. **A,** X-ray showing persistent displacement following nonoperative treatment of an acute unstable fracture of the scaphoid. Note the "ground glass" appearance of the bone in the proximal fragment suggestive of avascular necrosis. **B,** MRI of this patient showing a "black hole" (arrow) appearance reported as being indicative of avascular necrosis.

TREATMENT

When considering treatment, it is useful to compare avascular necrosis of the scaphoid with Kienböck's disease of the lunate.

Thus in the early stages of ischaemia (equivalent to stages I-II Kienböck's disease), treatment is aimed at reversing the pathological process before necrosis and collapse can occur.

Early Treatment

When x-ray films show signs suggestive of ischaemia of the proximal fragment after an acute scaphoid fracture, conservative treatment should be abandoned in favour of open reduction and *internal fixation with bone grafting* where appropriate. As the fracture heals, the radiological appearance of the bone should gradually return to normal (Figure 8-5). However, it may be at least 18 months before one can be confident that the bone is viable, so careful follow-up is essential.

Vascularised grafts may have a place in the management of ischaemia of the scaphoid, particularly in the early stages of Preiser's disease or when the proximal fragment appears completely ischaemic at the time of reconstructive surgery. If this technique can reverse early Kienböck's disease, there is no reason why it should not be applied successfully to the scaphoid as well. As yet, I have no personal experience with the use of vascularised bone grafts in scaphoid surgery. However, I would caution against volar pedicled grafts since these normally require prolonged immobilisation with the wrist in a flexed position and present a real risk of permanent stiffness. The experimental studies carried out by Hori et al.[2] suggest that successful revascularisation of bone requires the reestablishment of not only arterial supply but also venous drainage. Thus, a dorsal intermetacarpal arteriovenous pedicle, as described by Foucher and Saffar,[3] for lunate revascularisation may prove to be of some value in the treatment of the ischaemic scaphoid.

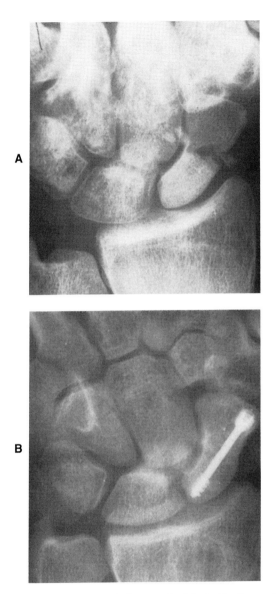

Figure 8-5. Reversible ischaemia of the scaphoid. **A,** Radiograph showing relative density of the proximal scaphoid fragment after plaster immobilisation of an acute unstable fracture. **B,** With bone grafting and screw fixation, the fracture has united and the density of both bone fragments now appears normal. (From Herbert TJ, Fisher WE. Management of the fractured scaphoid using a new bone screw. J Bone Joint Surg 66B:114, 1984.)

Chapter 8

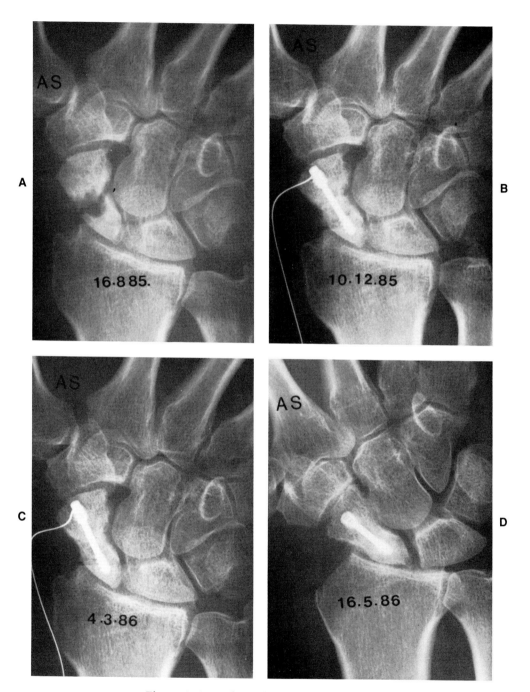

Figure 8-6. For legend see opposite page.

Figure 8-6. Radiographs of a patient who had a 3-year-old nonunion of the scaphoid after two previous bone grafting procedures. His wrist had been immobilised in a plaster cast for almost 24 months, and he had been unable to work this entire time. **A,** Shows an unstable pseudarthrosis of the scaphoid with an ischaemic proximal pole (stage 4). Note irregularity of the radial styloid following previous surgery. **B,** X-ray film after scaphoid reconstruction that involved excision of the pseudarthrosis, an iliac crest bone graft, and rigid internal fixation. Because the proximal fragment appeared completely ischaemic at surgery, an implanted bone growth stimulator was used. The lead is attached to the distal end of the screw. **C,** X-ray appearance of the scaphoid 3 months later; union appears complete, and the patient had been able to return to truck driving 1 month after surgery. **D,** The final appearance after a radial styloidectomy for symptoms caused by radiocarpal impingement. Note the improved range of radial deviation.

An alternative approach is to consider the use of a *bone growth stimulator*. I have been carrying out a clinical trial using a small implanted stimulator with a flexible electrode. Following internal fixation, the electrode is coupled to the screw using a small titanium plug that locks into the hexagonal socket (Figure 8-6). I have used this technique as an adjunct to reconstruction for a number of patients in whom the proximal pole appeared completely ischaemic at the time of surgery. Some of the fractures have united and some have not. On two separate occasions I have attached the stimulator some months after scaphoid reconstruction when there have been signs of impending nonunion. In neither case has this treatment appeared to make any difference. Although my total experience is limited, I doubt whether bone growth stimulation can favourably affect union rate in the presence of ischaemia.

Late Treatment

When the proximal pole of the scaphoid has undergone complete avascular necrosis, the changes are irreversible and reconstruction is no longer possible (equivalent to stage IV Kienböck's disease). Although the disease process may burn itself out eventually, carpal collapse deformity

Chapter 8

and secondary arthritis are almost inevitable and most patients require surgical treatment.

Removal of all necrotic bone and inflamed synovium normally produces rapid symptomatic relief. There is no need to remove the healthy distal pole of the scaphoid, which remains firmly attached to the adjacent bones and continues to impart some degree of stability to the wrist. For this reason, my preferred treatment for symptomatic avascular necrosis of the scaphoid is to carry out *prosthetic replacement of the proximal pole* only combined with a local synovectomy when necessary. As long as no associated midcarpal instability exists, this procedure provides excellent pain relief with improved range of motion and wrist function[4] and is preferable to the alternatives of *total scaphoid replacement, limited or total fusion,* or a *proximal row carpectomy.* Carter et

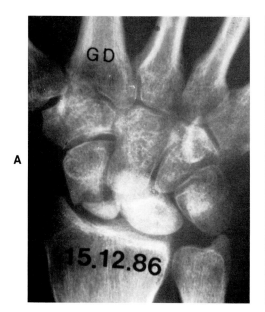
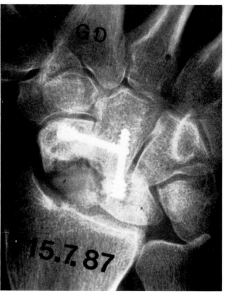

Figure 8-7. **A,** X-ray film of a patient with avascular necrosis of the proximal pole of the scaphoid together with severe carpal instability following prolonged plaster treatment of a transscaphoid-perilunate fracture dislocation. **B,** Postoperative x-ray appearance after partial Silastic replacement of the scaphoid. Limited intercarpal fusion was required to control instability. A very satisfactory clinical result was achieved with this patient.

al.[1] have recently reported encouraging short-term results using *allografts* to replace the proximal pole of the scaphoid. Although this is a fascinating clinical experiment, long-term follow-up is required before allografting can be universally recommended. In the meanwhile, I continue to treat patients by partial prosthetic replacement.

The most suitable prosthesis currently available is the Swanson Silastic scaphoid. This is a flexible implant that can be cut by hand and fashioned to the appropriate size and shape. It is essential to check the stability of the midcarpal joint before and at the time of the operation. Fortunately, most patients have a stable wrist with a fixed carpal collapse deformity secondary to long-standing nonunion of the scaphoid. However, in patients with ligamentous laxity or marked carpal instability, midcarpal fusion is mandatory when carrying out this procedure (Figure 8-7).

Preoperatively it may not be possible to decide whether the proximal fragment will be suitable for reconstruction or whether it needs to be replaced. The patient should be warned that the appropriate surgical procedure may need to be decided upon at the time of surgery.

PARTIAL SILASTIC REPLACEMENT
Surgical Technique (Figure 8-8)

Ideally partial Silastic replacement of the scaphoid should be carried out through the volar approach (Figure 8-8, *A*). However, in the case of a small proximal pole fracture, when a possibility of reconstruction remains or when midcarpal fusion may be necessary, it is better to use a dorsal approach.

Assuming that midcarpal fusion is not required, incise the volar wrist capsule and retract it in the normal manner (Figure 8-8, *B*). Remove the necrotic proximal fragment carefully by sharp dissection, together with any inflamed synovium. Avascular necrosis may involve only the volar half of the proximal fragment, although the entire proximal pole needs to be removed if it is to be replaced. Identify and cleanly divide the scapholunate ligament, taking care to avoid damage to the articular surfaces of the lunate, radius, and capitate. Check the stability of the midcarpal joint and reef the dorsal capsule if this is excessively lax.

Carry out an osteotomy through the waist of the scaphoid, perpendicular to the scaphoid's long axis, and angled slightly dorsally (Figure 8-8, *C*). Forcibly dorsiflex and ulnar deviate the wrist to obtain a good view of the distal bone face. Use a small osteotome or curette to cut a square or rectangular cavity in the medulla of the distal pole and deepen the cavity as far as possible (Figure 8-8, *D*). Soak a size 1 Swanson prosthesis in saline. Fashion the prosthesis to fit comfortably in the space created after excision of the proximal half of the scaphoid. Carefully carve a square peg out of the distal pole of the prosthesis, using a two-blade technique to ensure that the base of the peg is not weakened by cutting into it (Figure 8-8, *E*). Perform a trial reduction and make

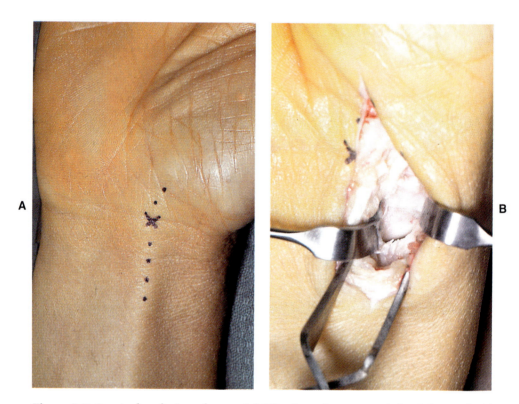

Figure 8-8. Surgical technique for partial Silastic replacement of the right scaphoid using the volar approach. **A,** Routine incision. **B,** Scaphoid exposed.

further adjustments as necessary. The peg should fit snugly within the cavity prepared in the distal pole and should impart sufficient stability to the prosthesis to prevent it from dislocating, even at the extremes of wrist movement (Figure 8-8, *F*).

Repair the volar wrist capsule with fine nonabsorbable sutures and check the range of motion and stability of the implant before closing the skin. Immobilise the wrist with a volar slab until the wound is healed. Provided the implant is stable at the time of surgery, gentle wrist exercises may be commenced, but the patient should avoid full extension and flexion for the first 6 weeks. Postoperative x-ray films should be taken to confirm satisfactory position of the prosthesis (Figure 8-8, *G*).

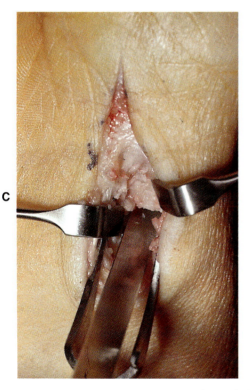
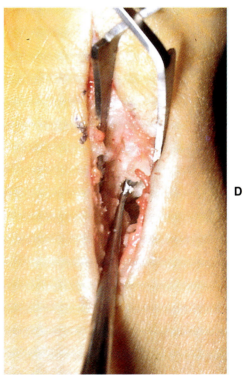

Figure 8-8, cont'd. C, Osteotomy through the distal waist; note that the cut is angled dorsally to increase stability. **D,** Shows cavity for the peg of the prosthesis being prepared in the distal fragment using a small curette. The wrist is in full dorsiflexion.

Continued.

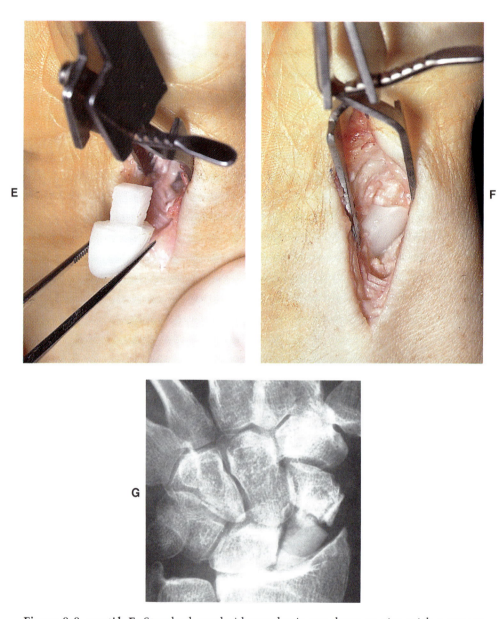

Figure 8-8, cont'd. E, Standard scaphoid prosthesis cut down to size with a square peg to lock into the distal fragment. **F,** Prosthesis inserted. Note the snug, stable fit. The wrist capsule is carefully repaired to prevent dislocation. **G,** Postoperative x-ray appearance after partial Silastic replacement of the scaphoid. Note the fit of the peg into the distal fragment.

When using the dorsal approach, it is more difficult to achieve stability of the implant. The dorsal wrist capsule should be reefed, and it is normally necessary to immobilise the wrist in dorsiflexion for a few weeks (Figure 8-9).

A check x-ray film is taken after 6 weeks. If the implant position remains satisfactory, the patient may resume normal activities. However, an elastic wrist support is advised for heavy labouring or contact sports. All patients are warned about the possibility of implant wear and the need for regular annual review to check for signs of silicone synovitis.

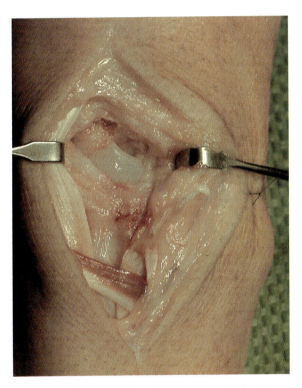

Figure 8-9. Intraoperative photograph to show partial Silastic replacement of the scaphoid carried out through a dorsal approach, right wrist. Note the snug fit of the prosthesis into the distal pole but the tendency to subluxate dorsally on wrist flexion. After careful repair of the dorsal capsule, the wrist was immobilised in dorsiflexion for 4 weeks.

Chapter 8

RESULTS AND COMPLICATIONS

Partial Silastic replacement of the scaphoid has been carried out in more than 80 patients, most of whom are young, active adults. The early results,[4] rapid pain relief and restoration of function, are encouraging. Most patients have been able to resume normal work and sporting activities, and I have been reassured by the amount of stress that they are able to withstand.

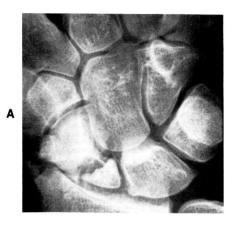

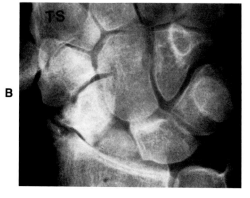

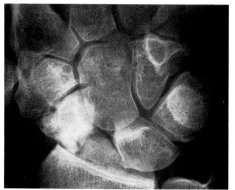

Figure 8-10. **A,** Preoperative x-ray film of a patient with long-standing nonunion of the scaphoid, following a failed Russe graft, with avascular necrosis of the proximal fragment and radiocarpal osteoarthritis secondary to impingement. **B,** Appearance after partial Silastic replacement of the scaphoid. **C,** Appearance after radial styloidectomy carried out 6 months later to relieve persistent radiocarpal impingement pain. The result was excellent.

The complications have included four cases of dislocation of the prosthesis, two early and two late. All of these appeared to be due to unrecognised instability of the midcarpal joint. Silicone synovitis has developed in six patients; again this problem appears to be related to unrecognised carpal instability with progressive collapse deformity, producing excessive loading on the prosthesis. The solution has been to remove the prosthesis and to carry out a midcarpal fusion combined with a local synovectomy.

Patients with significant radiocarpal osteoarthritis may continue to experience localised pain caused by radiocarpal impingement (Figure 8-10). This may be treated effectively by carrying out a limited radial styloidectomy (see Chapter 10).

The long-term prognosis following partial Silastic replacement remains uncertain, and I suspect that many of the patients will show signs of increasing implant wear and silicone synovitis. Clearly, a more suitable prosthesis is needed, but in the meantime the results of this procedure justify its use, even in young, active patients (Figure 8-11). If the prosthesis fails, it can always be revised using one of the alternative procedures outlined in the next chapter.

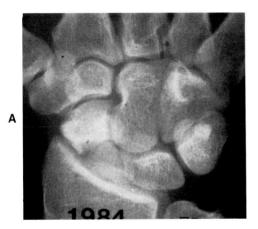
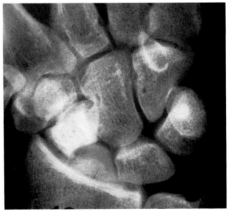

Figure 8-11. **A,** Radiographical appearance of the wrist after partial Silastic replacement of the scaphoid in a professional football player. **B,** X-ray film taken 3 years later shows some wear of the prosthesis. However, the patient has remained completely asymptomatic, has excellent wrist function, and has continued to play football. How long will the prosthesis last?

REFERENCES

1. Carter PR, Malinin TI, Abbey PA, Sommerkamp TG. The scaphoid allograft: A new operation for treatment of the very proximal scaphoid nonunion or for the necrotic, fragmented scaphoid proximal pole. J Hand Surg 14A:1, 1989.
2. Hori Y, Tamai S, Okuda H, Sakamoto H, Takita T, Masuhara K. Blood vessel transplantation to bone. J Hand Surg 4A:23-33, 1979.
3. Foucher G, Saffar PH. Revascularization of the necrosed lunate, stages I and II, with a dorsal intermetacarpal arteriovenous pedicle. J Chir Main 1:259, 1982.
4. Rath S, Herbert TJ. Hemisilastic replacement of scaphoid for avascular necrosis. Presented at the Fourth Congress of International Federation of Societies for Surgery of the Hand, Tel Aviv, April 1989.

9

Salvage Procedures for Scaphoid Nonunion

... Arthrodesis is the only certain way of achieving good pain relief, although in selected patients a number of other lesser procedures are worth considering.

Chapter 9

Most patients with a pseudarthrosis unsuitable for reconstruction can be managed conservatively, particularly when the demands on the wrist are not too great. Most middle-aged patients accept the advice that they should avoid overstraining the wrist and are prepared to wear an elastic wrist support when necessary. In younger, active patients with heavy demands on the wrist, arthrodesis is the only certain way of achieving good pain relief, although in selected patients a number of other lesser procedures are worth considering.

RADIAL STYLOIDECTOMY

As mentioned in Chapter 7, one of the aims of reconstructive surgery for scaphoid pseudarthrosis is to relieve pain arising from arthritic joints or osteophyte impingement. When arthritis is localised to the radiocarpal joint, symptoms are often relieved following reconstructive surgery, since lengthening the scaphoid with correction of the angulatory deformity prevents the distal fragment from impinging on the radius. In some patients with stage 4 pseudarthrosis in whom reconstruction of the scaphoid is contraindicated, a radial styloidectomy alone may be used to relieve symptoms associated with radiocarpal osteoarthritis.

In certain patients with radiocarpal arthritis, impingement may persist despite successful scaphoid reconstruction. Under these circumstances, symptoms may be relieved by excision of the radial styloid process (Figure 9-1). Characteristically these patients complain of pain on radial deviation and palmar flexion of the wrist, and both these movements may remain restricted. Although it may be tempting to consider carrying out a radial styloidectomy at the same time as scaphoid reconstruction, I prefer to wait at least 6 months after reconstruction before deciding whether a radial styloidectomy is indicated. A styloidectomy significantly increases the morbidity of reconstructive surgery and may affect wrist stability, preventing early postoperative mobilisation. At the same time, the temptation to use the radial styloid as the bone graft is avoided. In many patients with radiocarpal osteoarthritis, impingement will be relieved following reconstruction so that a styloidectomy is not required.

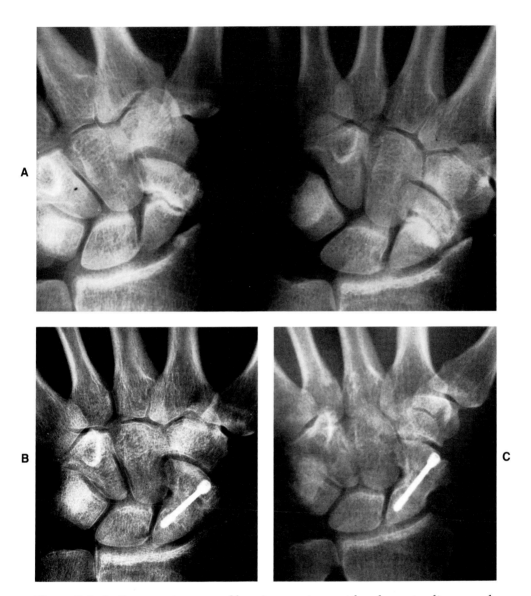

Figure 9-1. A, Preoperative x-ray films in a patient with a long-standing pseudarthrosis. Note the carpal collapse deformity with secondary radiocarpal arthritis. B, X-ray appearance after reconstruction using the standard technique of corticocancellous bone grafting with internal fixation. Although sound union was achieved, the patient had persistent symptoms caused by localised radiocarpal arthritis. C, Appearance after a radial styloidectomy and successful relief of symptoms.

Chapter 9

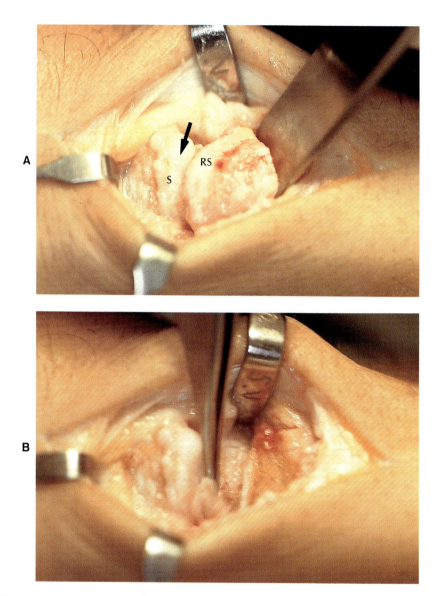

Figure 9-2. A, Operative photograph of radial styloidectomy, right wrist. Note impingement between the styloid (*RS*) and the dorsolateral osteophyte (arrow) on the scaphoid (*S*). **B,** Radiocarpal impingement has been relieved following removal of the styloid process; redundant synovium is here excised.

Operative Technique

Perform the operation through a longitudinal dorsoradial incision, taking care to protect the cutaneous branches of the radial nerve and the dorsal branch of the radial artery as it crosses the anatomical snuff-box. Incise the periosteum over the distal radius between the first and second extensor compartments and expose the bone subperiosteally. With the tendons retracted and the wrist held in ulnar deviation, use a fine osteotome to remove enough of the styloid process to relieve impingement on the distal part of the scaphoid when the wrist is radially deviated and palmar flexed (Figure 9-2). Examine the radiocarpal joint carefully and trim protruding osteophytes on the dorsum of the scaphoid. Plug the raw bone surface with bone wax, and repair the capsule and periosteum with fine, nonabsorbable sutures. The volar radiocarpal ligaments remain intact when this technique is used, so that instability is not a problem. However, a resting splint should be used for 2 to 3 weeks following the operation, after which time it is safe to mobilise the joint without further support.

OSTEOPHYTE EXCISION

In certain patients with stage 4 pseudarthrosis, pain relief may be achieved by simply excising prominent dorsal osteophytes, particularly if these are causing inflammation of the overlying soft tissues (Figure 9-3). Unfortunately, the osteophytes tend to recur unless the scaphoid has been stabilised. Because of this, I have occasionally carried out internal fixation of the fracture at the same time, without attempting to excise the pseudarthrosis or graft the fracture. I am not sure if this is a good idea, since stabilisation of the pseudarthrosis may restrict wrist motion. However, in one such patient with a long-standing proximal pole fracture (over 25 years) the improvement was dramatic, and x-ray films at 3 months appeared to show sound union of the fracture! I can offer no explanation for this phenomenon apart from the usual—that the radiograph should never be believed (Figure 9-4)!

Chapter 9

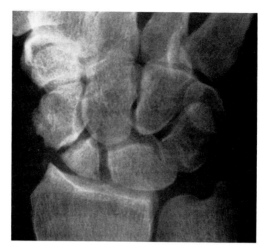

Figure 9-3. This middle-aged patient with a stage 4 scaphoid pseudarthrosis presented with a painful swelling on the back of the wrist caused by dorsal osteophytes. He was treated with a limited radial styloidectomy and excision of the dorsal osteophytes, with good symptomatic relief.

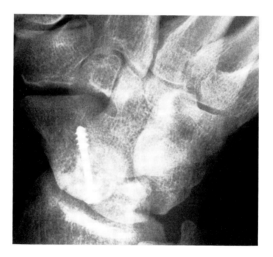

Figure 9-4. X-ray appearance 3 months postoperatively in a patient with osteoarthritis secondary to long-standing scaphoid pseudarthrosis. At operation, the dorsal osteophytes were removed and the fracture was stabilised by compression screw fixation. X-ray films suggest that the fracture may have healed in spite of the fact that no attempt was made to excise and graft it.

WRIST DENERVATION

I have no personal experience with this technique, although colleagues have reported significant pain relief in patients with arthritic wrists caused by long-standing scaphoid pseudarthrosis. However, the pain relief may be temporary, and many patients require further surgery.

The technique as first described by Wilhelm[1] and later in more detail by Buck-Gramcko[2] is a demanding one and requires as complete a denervation as possible. Provided that improvement can be maintained and no significant complications occur, I believe this procedure may be worth considering in selected patients.

SCAPHOID ARTHROPLASTY AND LIMITED INTERCARPAL FUSION

In selected patients with panscaphoid osteoarthritis total replacement of the scaphoid is worth considering.[3] Unless the midcarpal joint is stable and painless, however, this procedure should be combined with a fusion across the midcarpal joint (Figure 9-5). Without this fusion, progressive carpal subluxation is likely to occur, causing an overload on or dislocation of the prosthesis and a high risk of silicone synovitis (Figure 9-6, A to C).

Since many of these patients already have a long-standing carpal collapse deformity with secondary capitolunate osteoarthritis, the loss of motion after midcarpal fusion is unlikely to trouble the patient. However, at the time of fusion it is important to correct the midcarpal subluxation as much as possible in order to improve the range of dorsiflexion (Figure 9-6, D to F). Unless at least 30 degrees of extension are maintained after surgery, the patient will almost certainly continue to experience pain when the wrist is loaded. Young, active patients in particular are likely to complain of continued pain and functional impairment following limited intercarpal fusion, probably due to increased strain across adjacent unfused joints. Most of these patients prefer to have their wrists formally fused. However, in selected middle-aged patients with relatively low demands, Silastic replacement of the scaphoid combined with midcarpal fusion (SLAC procedure[4]) normally gives satisfactory results.

Chapter 9

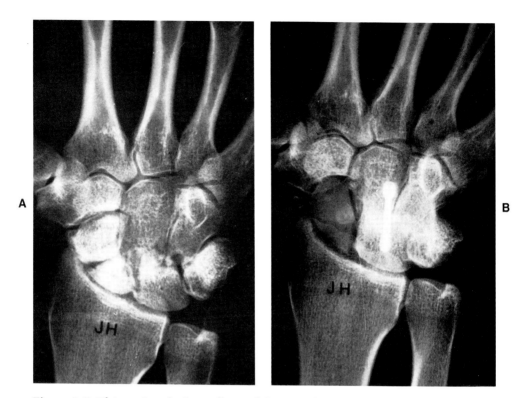

Figure 9-5. This patient had a stiff, painful wrist after conservative treatment for a transscaphoid-perilunate fracture dislocation of the carpus. **A,** X-ray film shows persistent nonunion with panscaphoid osteoarthritis and subluxation of the midcarpal joint. **B,** X-ray film after Silastic replacement of the scaphoid and midcarpal fusion. The patient's pain was relieved, but the range of motion remained restricted.

Figure 9-6. A, X-ray film taken in 1977, when a symptomatic scaphoid nonunion was diagnosed. The patient should have had a scaphoid reconstruction at this stage. **B,** X-ray film taken in 1979, after the patient had undergone total Silastic replacement of the scaphoid without midcarpal fusion. **C,** X-ray appearance 9 years later, when the patient sought treatment for increasing pain, swelling, and stiffness of the wrist. Note progression of midcarpal subluxation and secondary osteoarthritis. The cystic appearance of the capitate is highly suggestive of silicone synovitis.

Continued.

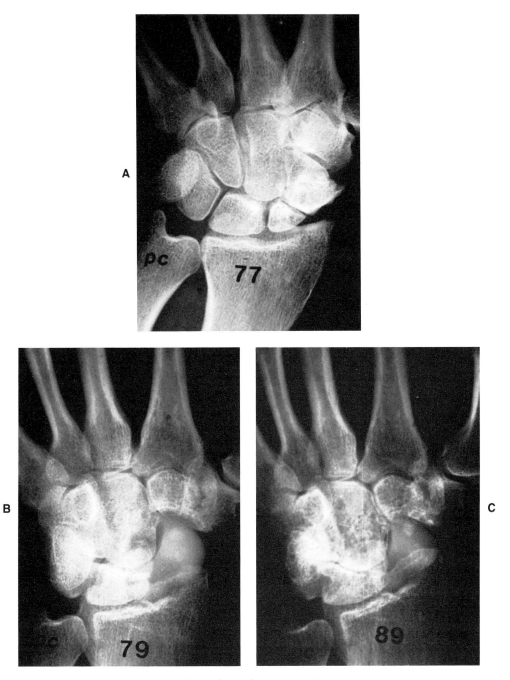

Figure 9-6. For legend see opposite page.

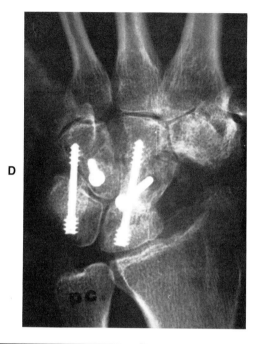

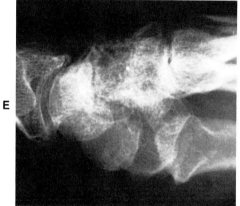
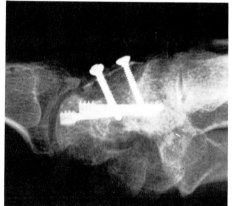

Figure 9-6, cont'd. D, X-ray appearance after removal of the prosthesis and synovectomy. The midcarpal subluxation has been reduced, internally fixed, and supplemented using an onlay bone graft technique. **E,** Preoperative lateral x-ray film shows the degree of carpal collapse deformity; extension of the wrist was limited to 10 degrees only. **F,** On the postoperative x-ray film midcarpal joint alignment is improved to the maximal degree that could be achieved. The wrist can now extend to 30 degrees. To obtain midcarpal fusion two Herbert screws were passed across the midcarpal joint to maintain the reduction. An onlay bone graft placed across the joint consolidated the fusion.

Operative Technique

Perform the procedure through a midline dorsal incision and divide the wrist capsule between the third and fourth extensor compartments. Excise the scaphoid in one piece by sharp dissection, taking care to avoid damage to the adjacent joint surfaces and to the wrist capsule. I prefer not to leave bone fragments behind because these may form painful osteophytes.

A size 1 Swanson scaphoid prosthesis is normally large enough and, indeed, may need to be trimmed before it will fit comfortably, particularly when the wrist is radially deviated. It is important not to "load" the prosthesis, since this greatly increases the risk of wear and silicone synovitis. Normally I try to stabilise the prosthesis by pegging it into the trapezium, but this is not always possible.

Examine the midcarpal joint for stability and arthritic changes and decide whether it should be fused. When fusing the joint, use a strong Kirschner wire as a lever to correct the dorsiflexion deformity of the lunate; once a satisfactory reduction has been achieved, pass a second Kirschner wire across the midcarpal joint from the capitate into the lunate, thus maintaining the alignment. Check extension of the wrist and if it does not reach 35 to 40 degrees, adjust the position of the wires. Fuse the midcarpal joint using an appropriate technique.

In the past I excised the joint surfaces completely and used interpositional bone grafts with internal fixation. However, this is a difficult procedure, and it is hard to maintain the correct position and avoid undue distortion of the unfused joints. I now prefer to leave the joint surfaces intact and rely on compression from one or more Herbert screws across the joint to achieve a stable synchondrosis. This is a relatively new technique and has not yet stood the test of time. Its simplicity is attractive, and it is quite simple to supplement the "fusion" with a dorsal onlay graft should this be considered necessary (Figure 9-6, *F*).

Chapter 9

PROXIMAL ROW CARPECTOMY

Excision of the scaphoid, lunate, and triquetrum has been championed for many years as a satisfactory solution to problems arising from a long-standing scaphoid nonunion.[5] I have been rather disappointed with the results of this procedure, although there is still considerable enthusiasm for it, particularly in the United States.[6] I believe a proximal row carpectomy should be considered only in patients with panscaphoid and midcarpal osteoarthritis who wish to retain some wrist motion at the expense of stability, pain relief, and power since relative lengthening of the flexor tendons may lead to some loss of grip strength.

Green[7] states that this procedure should not be carried out if arthritic changes involve the articular surface of the capitate. However, in this type of salvage procedure it is difficult to be so selective. I do not believe that capitate arthritis mitigates against a successful proximal row carpectomy, especially if a soft tissue interposition technique is used. If the patient is unhappy with the result, revision to fusion is fairly simple.

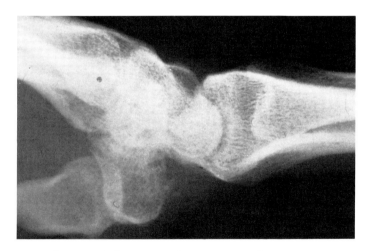

Figure 9-7. Lateral view of the wrist after a proximal row carpectomy. Note the satisfactory articulation between the proximal pole of the capitate and the distal articular surface of the radius.

Operative Technique

Carry out the operation through a midline dorsal approach, incising the capsule longitudinally between the third and fourth extensor compartments. Make a T-shaped extension to expose the triquetrum. Excise the triquetrum, lunate, and scaphoid by sharp dissection, taking care to avoid damaging the articular surfaces of the radius, ulna, and distal row bones. Wrist stability is improved by suturing redundant capsule and synovium between the capitate and the radius as a form of soft tissue interposition arthroplasty. Avoid transfixation wires and immobilise the wrist in a plaster cast for no longer than 6 weeks, after which the patient begins an exercise program (Figure 9-7).

WRIST FUSION

Arthrodesis of the wrist is probably the procedure of choice in younger patients with high functional demands in whom scaphoid reconstruction is not possible. These patients are usually disappointed with the results of all other salvage procedures. However, it is difficult to convince a patient to accept the idea of a wrist arthrodesis when the joint still has a reasonably good range of motion. Although in the first instance many of these patients may elect a "motion-preserving" procedure, the majority will end up requesting a wrist fusion.

The pain relief associated with a successful fusion results in significant improvement of hand function and grip strength. Unless special circumstances dictate otherwise, the wrist should be fused in 25 to 30 degrees of dorsiflexion, with neutral deviation.

Operative Technique

Use a straight midline dorsal incision extending from the midshaft of the middle metacarpal to the distal third of the radius. Divide the extensor retinaculum between the third and fourth compartments and elevate it from the radius so that it can later be repaired. Retract the extensor tendons and excise the joint surfaces of the distal radius and all carpal bones. Pack the resulting cavity with cancellous bone graft. Leave the carpometacarpal joints of the ulnar two digits undisturbed unless they are diseased. If the patient has undergone a previous Silastic arthroplasty, remove the prosthesis and fill the space with a block of cancellous bone.

Take a slab of corticocancellous bone from the outer border of the iliac crest. Lay the graft over the dorsum of the wrist and impact the graft into position with the wrist held in the appropriate degree of extension.

Internal fixation is achieved using a T-shaped plate with 3.5 mm cortical screws. Contour the plate to fit the bone and to hold the wrist in the correct position. Proximally, attach the plate to the radius using at least three screws; carefully curve the distal end of the plate over the bases of the second and third metacarpal bones and fix the plate to each of these using cortical screws of appropriate length (Figure 9-8).

The extensor carpi radialis brevis tendon may be detached from its insertion and sutured over the plate to cover the screw heads (Figure 9-9). Reposition the extensor pollicis longus and extensor digitorum

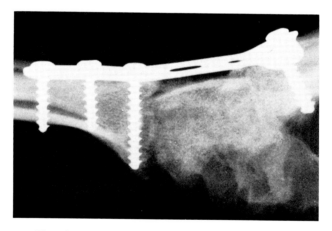

Figure 9-8. X-ray film shows technique of wrist fusion. A slab of corticocancellous bone graft has been firmly impacted between the radius and the base of the metacarpals. The plate has been contoured to hold the wrist in approximately 20 degrees of extension and has been fixed to the distal radius and to the shafts of the second and third metacarpals. (From Herbert TJ. Scaphoid fractures: Operative treatment. In Barton NJ, ed. Fractures of the Hand and Wrist. Edinburgh: Churchill Livingstone, 1988, p 234.)

communis tendons, and carefully repair the extensor retinaculum. Suction drainage is mandatory, and the wrist is protected in a light plaster cast for approximately 3 to 4 weeks. Remove the plate as soon as the fusion is sound, normally at 6 months. If required, carry out extensor tenolysis at the same time to ensure maximal recovery of hand function.

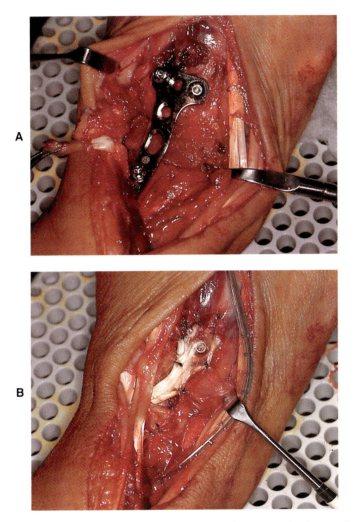

Figure 9-9. Intraoperative photograph after wrist fusion with plate and screw fixation (**A**) (hand toward top, forearm at bottom). The extensor carpi radialis brevis tendon has been detached and swung across to cover the plate and screws (**B**).

REFERENCES

1. Wilhelm K. Die Gelenkdenervation und Ihre Anatomischen Grundlagen. Ein Neues Behandlungsprinzip in der Handchirurgie. Hefte Unfallheik 86:1-109, 1966.
2. Buck-Gramcko D. Denervation of the wrist joint. J Hand Surg 2:54, 1977.
3. Vender MI, Watson HK, Black DM, Strickland JW. Acute scaphoid fracture with scapholunate gap. J Hand Surg 14A:1004, 1989.
4. Watson HK, Ballet FL. The SLAC wrist: Scapholunate advanced collapse pattern of degenerative arthritis. J Hand Surg 9A:358, 1984.
5. McLaughlin HL, Baab OD. Carpectomy. Surg Clin North Am 31:451, 1951.
6. Neviaser RJ. Proximal row carpectomy for posttraumatic disorders of the carpus. J Hand Surg 8:301, 1983.
7. Green D. Personal communication, 1987.

10

Scaphoid Malunion

... Corrective osteotomy of the scaphoid
will become an increasingly common operation
in future years.

Chapter 10

Malunion is a common, although seldom recognised, complication of scaphoid fractures. It does not rate a mention in the standard texts, and only recently has any reference been made to it in the literature.[1-3]

Malunion occurs following conservative treatment of unstable fractures of the body of the scaphoid, or after surgery, if anatomical reduction has not been achieved. Displaced fractures of the tubercle commonly result in malunion but only rarely cause problems (Figure 10-1).

The symptoms of malunion vary. Although many patients remain asymptomatic, some will complain of permanent loss of motion and pain on stressing the wrist. Scaphoid shortening usually restricts wrist extension, causing significant disability, particularly in young, physically active patients.

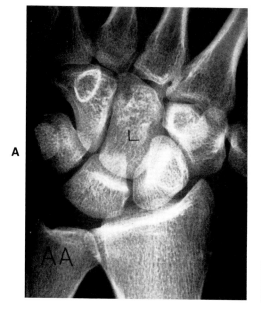 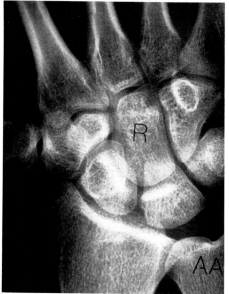

Figure 10-1. This patient experienced pain and restricted radial deviation of the right wrist after conservative treatment for a fracture of the scaphoid tubercle. **A,** X-ray appearance of the left uninjured wrist. Note the healthy joint space between the distal pole of the scaphoid and the radius. **B,** X-ray film of the right wrist showing reduced radiocarpal joint space and irregularity of the distal pole of the scaphoid.

Scaphoid Malunion

Scaphoid malunion also increases the risk of posttraumatic osteoarthritis, particularly when it is associated with a significant degree of carpal collapse deformity.

DIAGNOSIS

The diagnosis of malunion involves a high degree of awareness and careful comparison of the length and shape of the affected scaphoid with that of the opposite normal wrist (Figure 10-2). If significant shortening or anterior angulation of the scaphoid has occurred, the lateral x-ray films will show a corresponding degree of carpal collapse deformity (Figure 10-3).

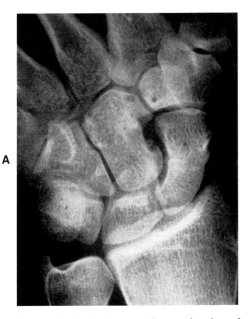
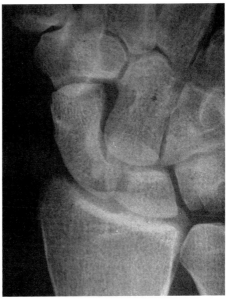

Figure 10-2. Patient with scaphoid malunion after conservative treatment of an acute fracture. The patient presented at 1 year with persistent pain and loss of motion in the left wrist (**A**). Comparison with the opposite normal wrist (**B**) shows that the scaphoid is significantly shorter (malunion), and the displaced distal pole appears to be eroding the capitate.

Chapter 10

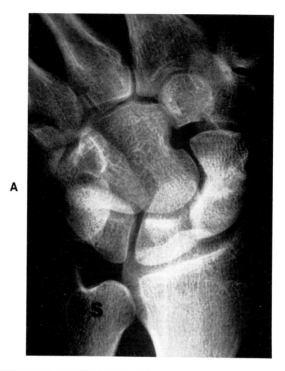

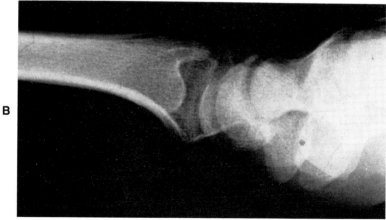

Figure 10-3. This patient had symptomatic malunion of the scaphoid after treatment in a plaster cast for an acute fracture. Wrist extension was limited to 55 degrees with pain on stressing. **A,** Posteroanterior view showing deformity of the scaphoid. **B,** Lateral view showing associated carpal collapse deformity (DISI pattern) responsible for loss of wrist extension.

MANAGEMENT

Malunion of the scaphoid is best avoided by more aggressive treatment of the acute unstable fracture. If the patient is asymptomatic, reconstructive surgery is probably not justified unless long-term studies show that malunion will inevitably lead to disabling osteoarthritis.

However, I am seeing an increasing number of patients in whom malunion appears to be the cause of persistent disability. Under these circumstances I believe that *corrective osteotomy* of the scaphoid is a justifiable procedure in the management of symptomatic malunion in adults.

SURGICAL TECHNIQUE

Perform a careful preoperative assessment and measure the x-ray films to determine the degree of correction required.

Make a standard volar incision and, regardless of the level of the original fracture, carry out a transverse osteotomy through the scaphoid waist, perpendicular to the long axis of the bone. Force the wrist into full extension and wedge the osteotomy open as appropriate (Figure 10-4). If a lateral angulatory or rotatory deformity has occurred, attempt to correct the deformity by using temporary Kirschner wires as levers to control the bone fragments.

Obtain a corticocancellous bone graft from the iliac crest and carefully fashion the bone to fit tightly within the defect to maintain the correction. Internally fix the scaphoid and graft in the corrected position.

With rigid internal fixation, postoperative splinting is unnecessary and the patient can return to work within a few weeks of surgery.

Chapter 10

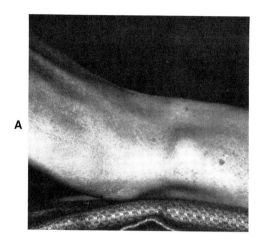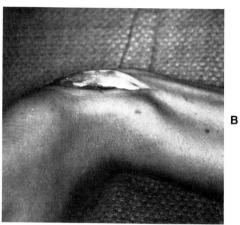

Figure 10-4. Same patient whose x-ray films are shown in Figure 10-3. **A,** Preoperative photograph demonstrating limited wrist extension. **B,** Intraoperative photograph showing improved extension following scaphoid osteotomy and bone grafting.

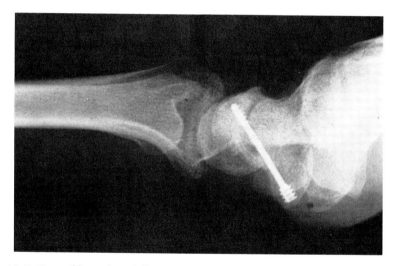

Figure 10-5. X-ray film taken following scaphoid osteotomy. Note correction of the previous carpal collapse deformity shown in Figure 10-3, *B*. This patient had an excellent clinical result, and the osteotomy was soundly healed after 6 weeks. No postoperative casting was required.

RESULTS AND COMPLICATIONS

I have not yet had sufficient experience to report the long-term results of this procedure. However, in the short term, notable improvements in wrist motion and pain relief have been achieved, and patients have been happy with the results of surgery. Postoperative x-ray films have shown significant improvement, but in only one case could it be said that normal anatomical alignment had been restored (Figure 10-5). Despite this, it is hoped that this procedure will improve the long-term prognosis and reduce the risk of osteoarthritis. For this reason, I believe that a corrective osteotomy of the scaphoid will become an increasingly common operation in future years.

REFERENCES

1. Herbert TJ, Fisher WE. Management of the fractured scaphoid using a new bone screw. J Bone Joint Surg 1B:114-123, 1984.
2. Amadio PC, Berquist TH, Smith DK, Ilstrup DM, Cooney WP, Linscheid RL. Scaphoid malunion. J Hand Surg 14A:679-687, 1989.
3. Nakamura R, Hori M, Horii E, Miura T. Reduction of the scaphoid fracture with DISI alignment. J Hand Surg 12A:1000-1005, 1987.

11

Scaphoid Fractures in the Skeletally Immature

... Diagnosis depends on an increased awareness of the possibility of scaphoid fractures in children. ...

Fractures of the tubercle are relatively common in children and may be treated as soft tissue injuries. Fractures of the waist of the scaphoid are rarely diagnosed, and nonunion is believed to be extremely uncommon.[1,2] Experience leads me to suspect that this may not be the case. Diagnosing an acute scaphoid fracture in children can be extremely difficult. The injury results from a simple fall and is easy to pass off as a "sprained wrist." X-ray films frequently fail to demonstrate the acute fracture (Figure 11-1). This may be because the fracture is incomplete, similar to a greenstick fracture in the forearm.

Most of the scaphoid fractures I have seen in the skeletally immature present as an established nonunion. Symptoms are frequently minimal and rarely do children have significant loss of motion. Presumably the ligamentous laxity of youth preserves a degree of function that belies the marked carpal collapse deformity and scaphoid shortening commonly found on x-ray films (Figure 11-2).

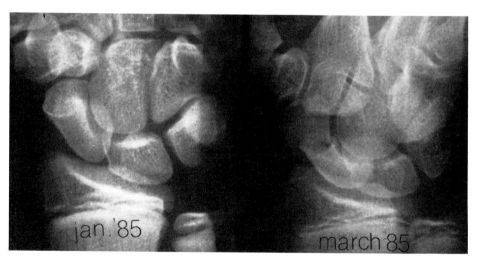

Figure 11-1. This 15-year-old boy sustained an acute scaphoid fracture in January 1985. The initial x-ray film showed no obvious fracture. However, despite prompt immobilisation of the wrist in a plaster cast, x-ray films taken at the time of cast removal 6 weeks later showed the development of a pseudarthrosis with associated carpal instability. (From Herbert TJ. Scaphoid fractures: Operative treatment. In Barton NJ, ed. Fractures of the Hand and Wrist. Edinburgh: Churchill Livingstone, 1988, p 221.)

Scaphoid Fractures in the Skeletally Immature

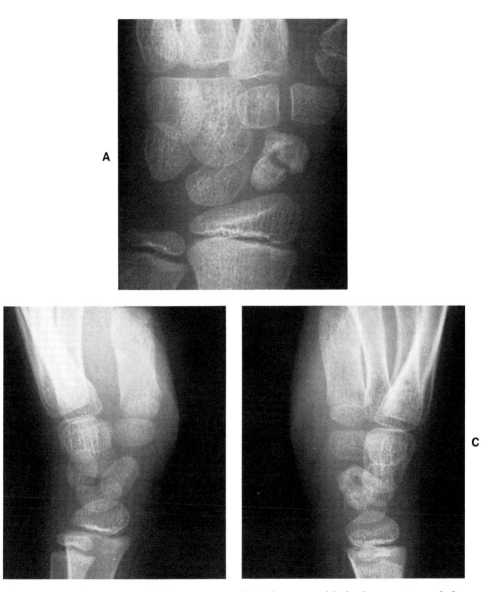

Figure 11-2. This 9-year-old boy presented with an established nonunion of the scaphoid. One year previously his wrist had been immobilised in a plaster cast for several weeks for a suspected scaphoid fracture. A, Posteroanterior view shows a typical nonunion with cystic change and a carpal collapse deformity. B and C, Lateral x-ray films of both wrists confirm the presence of a marked carpal collapse deformity associated with an unstable nonunion of the left scaphoid (C).

Chapter 11

DIAGNOSIS

The diagnosis depends on an increased awareness of the possibility of scaphoid fractures in children and careful follow-up in those diagnosed as having wrist sprains.

MANAGEMENT

If any doubt exists as to whether a child has sustained a scaphoid fracture, the wrist should be immobilised in a Colles'-type plaster cast for at least 4 weeks. Careful follow-up is essential, with a check x-ray examination performed after 1 year. Just as in adults, it can be difficult to determine from the x-ray appearance whether or not the fracture has united (Figure 11-3).

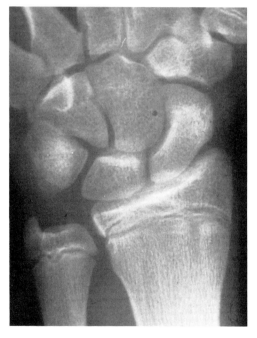

Figure 11-3. X-ray appearance after conservative treatment of an acute scaphoid fracture in a 14-year-old boy. Can we be certain that this fracture is united? Review at 1 year is recommended.

Scaphoid Fractures in the Skeletally Immature

The treatment of an established nonunion involves bone grafting and correction of any associated carpal collapse deformity. Because of the small size of the bone and to reduce the possibility of inhibiting growth or damaging the adjacent joints, I prefer to avoid screw fixation in children. It is better to immobilise the fracture with Kirschner wires and plaster (Figure 11-4). Fortunately, prolonged immobilisation of the wrist in children does not seem to cause any problems. Joint stiffness recovers rapidly and healing of the fracture is virtually guaranteed. The only disadvantage with Kirschner wires is that a second surgical procedure is required to remove them once the fracture has united.

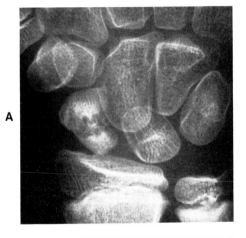
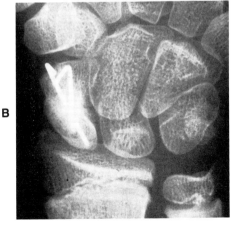

Figure 11-4. Established nonunion of the scaphoid in a 12-year-old child treated by bone grafting and internal fixation using Kirschner wires. **A,** Preoperative x-ray film showing nonunion with collapse. **B,** Postoperative x-ray appearance after removal of the plaster cast 2 months later. The fracture appears soundly united, with good correction of the collapse deformity. The patient required a subsequent procedure to remove the wires.

Small proximal pole fractures occasionally occur in the skeletally immature and often present with signs suggestive of avascular necrosis (Figure 11-5). This poses considerable problems in management. Whatever the radiological appearance, an attempt should be made to obtain healing by means of bone grafting. If left untreated, the prognosis is poor. Silastic arthroplasty is obviously contraindicated in this age group.

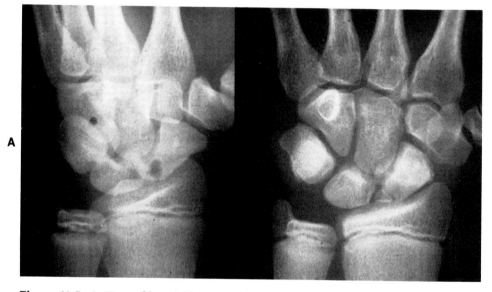

Figure 11-5. A, X-ray films (oblique and posteroanterior) of a 15-year-old boy who presented with established nonunion after a missed fracture through the proximal pole of the scaphoid. Although he was relatively asymptomatic, the x-ray appearance suggests that the proximal pole is undergoing avascular necrosis. What would you do in this case? **B,** The fracture was exposed and grafted through a direct dorsal incision. Fortunately, sufficient viable bone remained in the proximal fragment for it to be reattached with a Herbert screw. The x-ray appearance at 8 weeks is worrisome because of apparent resorption of the graft. **C,** X-ray films taken 4 months after surgery show that the fracture is now united, and the appearance of the proximal pole is improving. The screw was later removed and the patient made an uneventful recovery.

Scaphoid Fractures in the Skeletally Immature

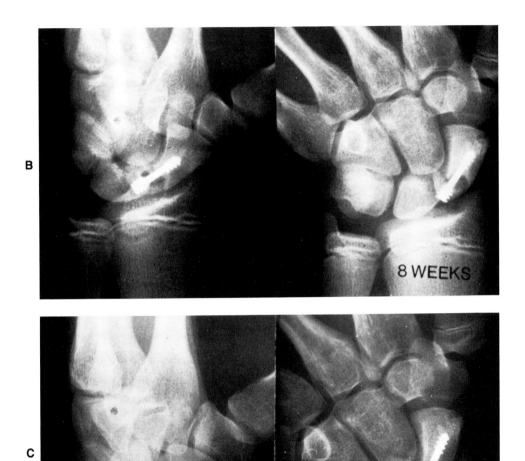

Figure 11-5, cont'd. For legend see opposite page.

Chapter 11

COMPLICATIONS

I have seen two children with severe *malunion* of the scaphoid, one after conservative treatment and the other after bone grafting. Both of these children remain under regular review, and I have been pleased to observe steady correction of the deformity (Figure 11-6). My recommendation is to delay consideration of corrective osteotomy until the patient has reached skeletal maturity.

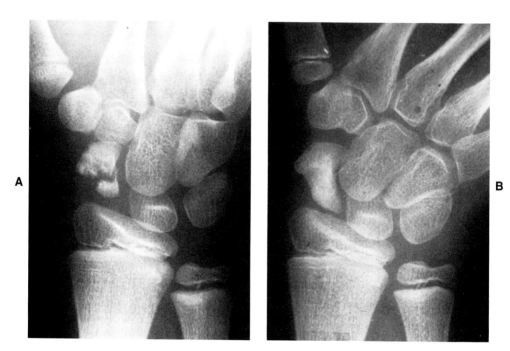

Figure 11-6. Malunion of the scaphoid in a child. **A,** Symptomatic nonunion in a child. **B,** X-ray appearance showing union following Russe-type bone grafting procedure. Note, however, the irregular appearance of the scaphoid.

Scaphoid Fractures in the Skeletally Immature

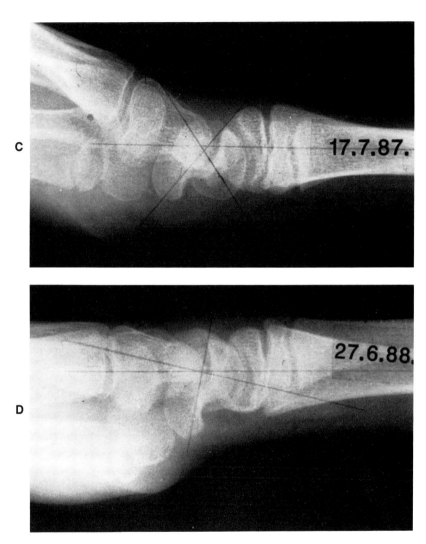

Figure 11-6, cont'd. C, Lateral x-ray film confirms malunion of the scaphoid with severe carpal collapse deformity. **D,** X-ray appearance 1 year later shows marked improvement in the carpal alignment, presumably because of scaphoid remodelling with growth.

REFERENCES

1. Vahvanen V, Westerlund M. Fracture of the carpal scaphoid in children. Acta Orthop Scand 51:909, 1980.
2. Southcott R, Rosman MA. Nonunion of carpal scaphoid fractures in children. J Bone Joint Surg 59B:20, 1977.

12

Rotary Subluxation of the Scaphoid

It is vital that this condition be diagnosed and treated promptly.

Chapter 12

The scaphoid bone is the keystone of the wrist. It has already been demonstrated that stability of the midcarpal joint depends on an intact "scaphoid link" (Figure 12-1). When the midcarpal joint is subjected to a major deforming force, this link may fail because of a scaphoid fracture or a rupture of the ligaments that support it (Figure 12-2). When a ligament rupture occurs, the carpus becomes unstable. The scaphoid tends to rotate into an anteverted position, whereas the lunate and triquetrum subluxate volarly, producing the DISI deformity.

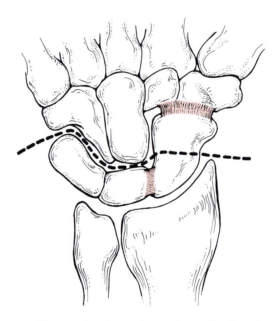

Figure 12-1. The scaphoid bone "bridges" the midcarpal joint. Because of its strong proximal and distal ligamentous attachments, the bone acts as a restraining link, preventing dislocation of the midcarpal joint. The dotted line shows how the stress axis of the midcarpal joint passes across the scaphoid waist.

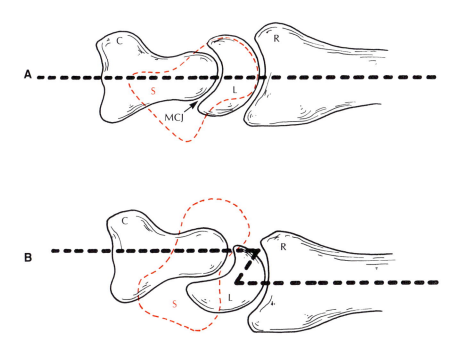

Figure 12-2. A, The scaphoid bone (S) by means of its proximal attachment to the lunate (L) and distal attachment to the capitate (C) acts as a link to support the midcarpal joint (MCJ). R, radius. **B,** With rupture of the scapholunate ligament, the scaphoid tends to assume a flexed, or anteverted, position, allowing the carpus to collapse. (Modified from Fisk GR. Carpal instability and the fractured scaphoid. Ann Roy Coll Surg Engl 46:63, 1970.)

The degree of deformity depends on the severity of the initial trauma, and the clinical picture may range from complete dislocation to a subtle form of dynamic instability.

However, once the supporting link has been weakened, repeated movement and stress across the midcarpal joint cause progressive subluxation and osteoarthritic changes at both the radioscaphoid and midcarpal joints. Because of the nature of the deformity, irreversible changes may occur within a few months of injury (Figure 12-3). It is vital that this condition be diagnosed and treated promptly.

As with scaphoid fractures, not all patients have a classic history of injury. At one end of the spectrum are patients who cannot recall any significant injury but who have symptoms and signs of dynamic instability. These patients are usually young women with generalised ligament laxity. At the other extreme are patients with chronic rotary dislocation of the scaphoid. This condition is starting to be recognised as the cause of symptomatic osteoarthritis of the wrist in middle-aged men who have engaged in heavy manual work over many years. In some patients the dislocation is obviously of long standing, whereas in others it occurs after relatively minor trauma in a wrist already affected by osteoarthritis. In a third group of patients, acute rotary dislocation of the scaphoid is clearly the result of major trauma in which other injuries (e.g., radial styloid fractures) may also occur. For this reason, I find it useful to classify rotary subluxation of the scaphoid as follows:

Type 1: Dynamic: Dynamic instability typically occurs in young women with ligamentous laxity and results from relatively minor trauma (Figure 12-4).

Type 2: Static: Rotary dislocation of the scaphoid results from ligamentous disruption following major trauma. It appears to occur exclusively in young men (Figure 12-5).

Type 3: Arthritic: Chronic rotary subluxation of the scaphoid is commonly seen in patients with osteoarthritis of the wrist and attrition rupture of the scapholunate ligament. It is usually bilateral and tends to occur in middle-aged men who have subjected the wrist to heavy or repetitive strains over many years. It is surprisingly common in golfers (Figure 12-6).

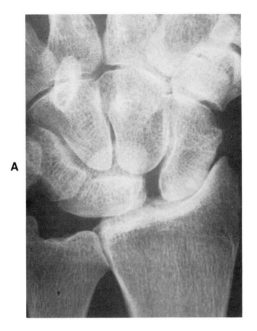
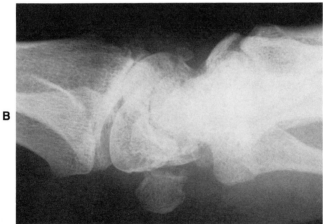

Figure 12-3. X-ray appearance 18 months after an untreated scapholunate ligament rupture. **A,** The posteroanterior view shows almost complete loss of normal joint space between the scaphoid and the radius. **B,** In the lateral x-ray film the proximal pole of the scaphoid may be seen impinging on the dorsal lip of the radius, leading to the rapid development of osteoarthritis. Note also the avulsion fracture of the dorsum of the scaphoid. This is a common finding with a scapholunate ligament injury.

Chapter 12

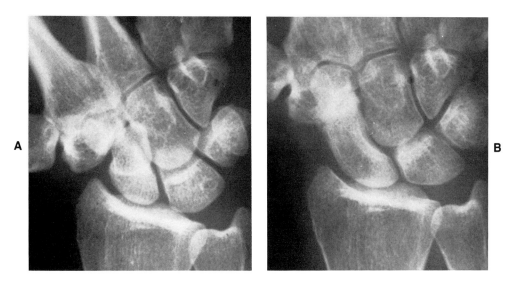

Figure 12-4. Type 1: dynamic. **A,** Stress x-ray film shows a dynamic instability of the scaphoid in a young female athlete. The scapholunate ligament is intact. **B,** X-ray appearance after STT fusion, which successfully relieved the patient's symptoms but left her with significant loss of wrist extension.

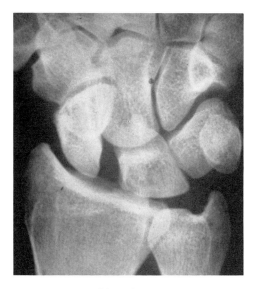

Figure 12-5. Type 2: static. X-ray film shows an acute rotary dislocation of the scaphoid after a major hyperextension injury of the wrist. This condition occurs exclusively in young adult men.

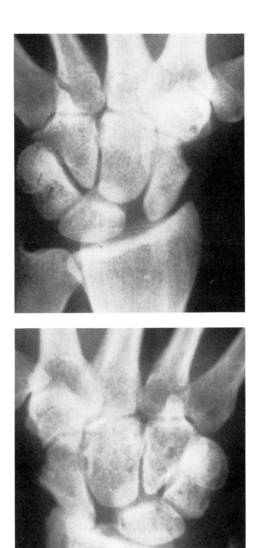

Figure 12-6. Type 3: arthritic. This 48-year-old man had symptoms of osteoarthritis in the right wrist. X-ray films show signs of bilateral rupture of the scapholunate ligaments. Secondary degenerative changes are more advanced on the right side. This patient was unable to recall any episode of acute trauma but had subjected his wrists to constant overloading through the use of heavy shifters in his work as a fitter and turner.

DIAGNOSIS
History

Diagnosis of rotary instability requires a high degree of awareness on the part of the surgeon and an accurate patient history. An acute dislocation (type 2) should be suspected in all patients with a history of significant trauma to the wrist but in whom a scaphoid fracture cannot be demonstrated. Patients with dynamic instability (type 1) complain of intermittent attacks of sharp pain associated with a sensation of "giving way" when the wrist is subjected to stress loading. Painful "locking" may also result from subluxation of the proximal pole of the scaphoid over the dorsal rim of the radius. Patients with type 3 rotary subluxation of the scaphoid often give a history of chronic wrist pain with increasing stiffness and weakness. Sometimes a relatively minor episode of trauma, such as mis-hitting a golf ball, produces an acute deterioration, presumably indicating complete rupture of the previously attenuated ligaments supporting the scaphoid.

Clinical Examination

In rotary subluxation the area of maximal tenderness is usually localised to the scapholunate junction on the dorsum of the wrist. Bimanual examination of the scaphoid may confirm the presence of abnormal anteversion (Figure 12-7), and it is sometimes possible to demonstrate instability by applying stress to the midcarpal joint. Similarly, it may be possible to feel the proximal pole of the scaphoid subluxate over the dorsal rim of the radius when the wrist is moved from full ulnar into full radial deviation, producing a palpable and audible "clunk."

Most patients experience significant functional impairment that can be measured by loss of grip strength.

Investigations

It may be surprisingly difficult to demonstrate any abnormality on plain x-ray films unless a fixed deformity has developed. Scapholunate diastasis is an unreliable sign, although the lateral view should confirm a vertically rotated scaphoid and dorsiflexion deformity of the

Rotary Subluxation of the Scaphoid

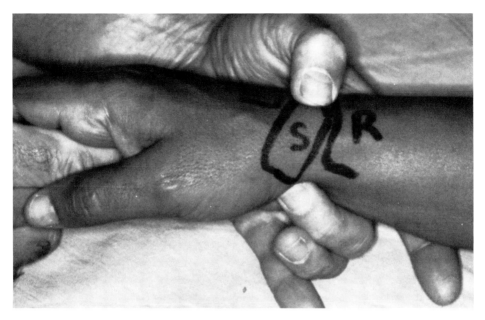

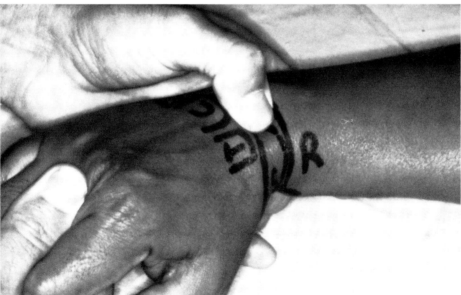

Figure 12-7. Careful palpation of the scaphoid whilst moving the wrist from ulnar to radial deviation reveals an abnormal degree of anteversion (rotary subluxation). Note how the examiner's thumb palpates the dorsal pole of the scaphoid whilst his middle finger presses firmly against the tubercle on the front of the wrist.

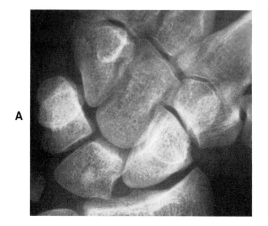 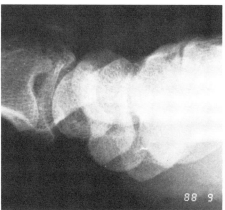

Figure 12-8. X-ray film of a patient with rotary dislocation of the scaphoid following carpal collapse deformity associated with ligamentous rupture of the scapholunate ligament. **A,** In the posteroanterior view there is no obvious scapholunate diastasis, although the bone appears foreshortened. **B,** The rotary dislocation of the scaphoid is best appreciated on the lateral x-ray film.

lunate, with subluxation of the midcarpal joint (Figure 12-8). However, the scaphoid normally appears foreshortened on the posteroanterior view, especially when compared with the opposite, uninjured side (Figure 12-9). In type 3 cases, x-ray films invariably show some degree of radiocarpal arthritis (see Figure 12-6).

Arthrography might be expected to confirm the diagnosis in all cases of scapholunate ligament rupture. However, this investigation tends to be unreliable, since posttraumatic adhesions may prevent a leak from occurring. Conversely, it is extremely common for intercarpal leaks to occur in a clinically normal wrist. Thus a positive arthrogram is only of diagnostic significance if simultaneous arthrography of the opposite, uninjured wrist is negative[1] (Figure 12-10).

Scintigraphy is not particularly helpful in diagnosing this condition, since the scan may be negative in the presence of a major ligament injury but positive in a wide variety of posttraumatic conditions. I have no experience in the use of tomography, CT, or MRI in the diagnosis of rotary subluxation of the scaphoid.

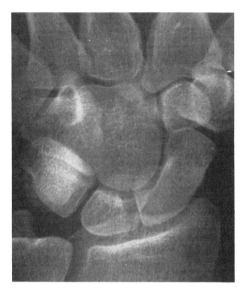 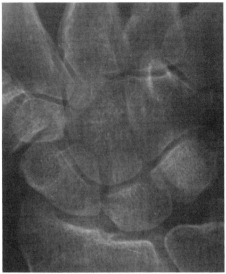

Figure 12-9. Posteroanterior view of both wrists shows foreshortening of the right scaphoid caused by rotary subluxation. The diagnosis was missed until comparative x-ray films of the opposite wrist were taken, by which time the dislocation was irreducible because of prolonged immobilisation in a plaster cast for the associated radial styloid fracture. This case represents a common diagnostic pitfall.

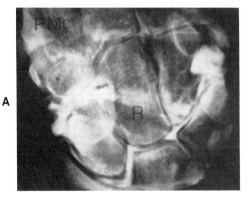 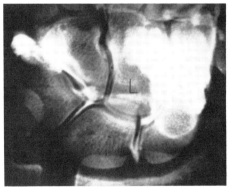

Figure 12-10. Midcarpal arthrography of the wrist. Note a significant leak of dye through the right scapholunate joint (**A**). This is a common finding in clinically normal wrists and is of significance only if a similar examination of the opposite asymptomatic wrist is negative (**B**). (From Herbert TJ, Faithfull RG, McCann DJ, Ireland J. Bilateral arthrography of the wrist. J Hand Surg 15B:233, 1990.)

Arthroscopy

Arthroscopy of the wrist is extremely useful in assessing the degree of deformity and the status of the ligaments and articular cartilage. However, arthroscopy is not indicated for acute dislocations (type 2) since urgent reconstructive surgery is required. Arthroscopic examination of the wrist is useful in patients with type 3 subluxations so that the appropriate surgical procedure can be planned, depending on the extent and degree of arthritis present.

MANAGEMENT

Management depends on the age of the patient, the degree of disability, and the type of subluxation.

Type 1: Dynamic Instability

Patients with dynamic instability should usually be managed conservatively, with the use of an elastic wrist support and suitable modification of activities. Occasionally symptoms are sufficiently troublesome, particularly in athletes, to warrant surgical treatment. I carry out a dorsal arthrotomy and then proceed either to capsulorrhaphy,[2] or to scapho-trapezial-trapezoid (STT) fusion,[3] depending on the degree of instability and the state of the joints (see Figure 12-4).

Type 2: Rotary Dislocation

Reconstructive surgery is indicated in all cases of acute dislocation. The sooner this is done the better, since irreversible damage to the articular cartilage may occur within a few weeks of injury.

SURGICAL TECHNIQUE (Figure 12-11)

Perform a dorsal arthrotomy and insert strong Kirschner wires into the lunate and scaphoid as levers to reduce the dislocation and to restore normal anatomical alignment. Blunt dissection may be required to free any intra-articular adhesions preventing reduction of the scaphoid or the lunate. Decide how best to hold the reduction. If possible, avoid intercarpal fusion, since this results in permanent loss of wrist motion. In contrast, a successful soft tissue repair may result in full recovery of wrist function.

I prefer to use fine, nonabsorbable sutures to repair or reattach the scapholunate ligament. If an avulsion fracture of the scaphoid or

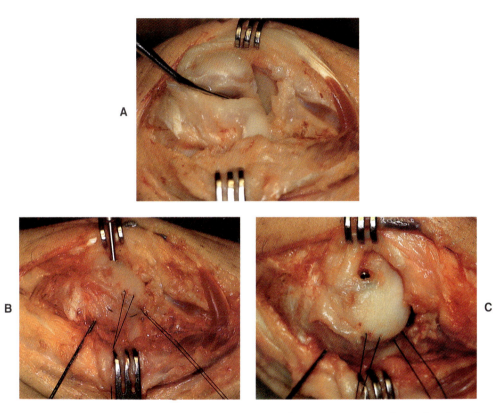

Figure 12-11. Operative repair of a scapholunate ligament rupture through a dorsal incision (right wrist, hand to left). **A,** Probe lies in the scapholunate joint. The ligament has been completely avulsed from the scaphoid, allowing it to rotate with dorsal dislocation of the proximal pole. **B,** The dislocation has been reduced and held with temporary Kirschner wires. The scapholunate ligament has been reattached to the scaphoid using nonabsorbable sutures passed through small drill holes in the bone. **C,** A Herbert screw has been inserted across the scapholunate joint to protect the ligament repair. The Kirschner wires were removed, and the patient was treated with early protected mobilisation of the wrist.

lunate is present, reattach the bone fragment. I have not as yet attempted to repair the volar radiocarpal ligaments, since such a repair would involve opening the front of the wrist as well as the back; nevertheless, I believe this approach may be worth considering.

The repair will need to be protected by some form of temporary internal fixation. The simplest method is to pass Kirschner wires across the scaphocapitate and scapholunate joints. The problem with this method is that the wires must be left protruding and may bend or break if any movement of the wrist is allowed. This means that immobilisation in a plaster cast must be continued for a considerable time, since these ligament injuries take many months to heal. Even after several months, the dislocation tends to recur when the wires are removed. For this reason, I now protect the repair by transfixing the scapholunate joint with a Herbert screw (Figure 12-12). The screw is inserted by the freehand method after first using a Kirschner wire across the joint to hold the reduction. The wire may be cut short and left in, providing two-point fixation, which helps to ensure a stable repair. Occasionally, the

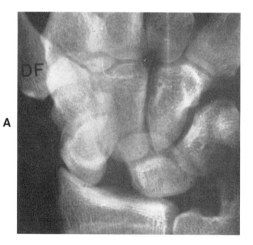
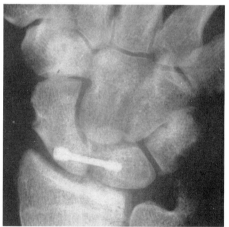

Figure 12-12. **A,** Preoperative x-ray in a patient with acute rotary dislocation of the scaphoid with complete rupture of the scapholunate ligament. **B,** After open reduction and ligament repair, a Herbert screw has been used to hold the reduction and protect the repair, at the same time allowing protected joint motion. (From Herbert TJ. Internal fixation of the carpus with the Herbert bone screw system. J Hand Surg 14A(2)(Part 2):397, 1989.)

scaphocapitate joint must also be pinned to hold a stable reduction, but I prefer to avoid this if possible.

I have been encouraged by the early results using this technique, since prolonged immobilisation is not required. Protected joint motion using a limited-motion wrist splint is commenced after a few days. Wrist motion remains restricted for as long as the scapholunate joint remains fixed. However, with increasing motion, the screw loosens in the bone, although it still provides some protection to the repair (Figure 12-13). Once loosening of the screw occurs, it is normally removed, since there

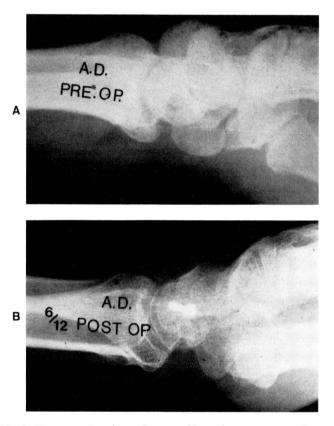

Figure 12-13. **A,** Preoperative lateral x-ray film of a patient with an acute rotary dislocation of the scaphoid that was treated by ligament repair and screw fixation. **B,** Six months later the scaphoid remains in normal alignment and the screw is starting to loosen.

Chapter 12

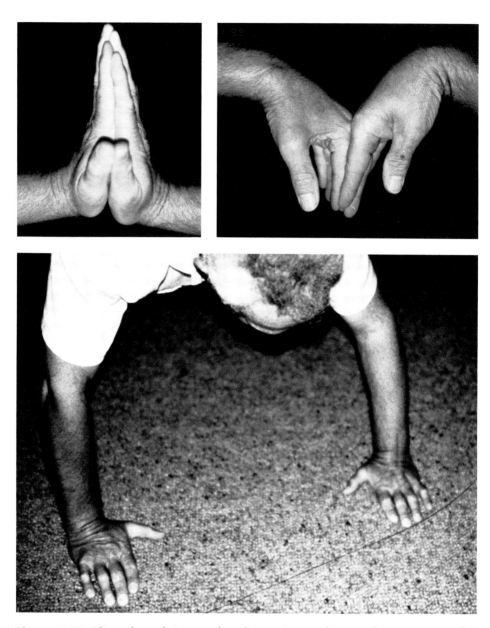

Figure 12-14. Clinical result 1 year after this patient underwent ligament repair for an acute rotary dislocation of the scaphoid in the right wrist. Note the almost full range of wrist extension but limited flexion. The patient can do a push-up without difficulty and returned to his job as a painter 6 weeks after the injury. To date, the screw has not been removed.

is otherwise a risk of breaking the implant or damaging the scaphoid or lunate. In a few cases there has been some recurrence of the deformity. However, in the majority the carpus has remained stable, with very satisfactory results (Figure 12-14).

I should point out that this is an extremely difficult surgical procedure, and the long-term results are not yet known. In one patient the deformity recurred following removal of the screw; in the remainder the carpus has remained stable and to date no deformity has recurred. It is too early to know whether this improvement will be maintained indefinitely (Figure 12-14).

Type 3: Arthritis

Patients with chronic rotary subluxation of the scaphoid should be managed conservatively whenever possible. An elastic wrist support provides considerable symptomatic relief, and the patient should be advised to avoid overstraining the wrist.

STT fusion is contraindicated in the presence of significant radiocarpal arthritis. Although the *SLAC* procedure described by Watson, Goodman, and Johnson[4] appears to offer a satisfactory solution, I have been disappointed with the results of this procedure in high-demand patients.

I have no experience with *wrist denervation*, although this seems a reasonable option to consider.

Wrist fusion offers the most certain solution, but most patients are unwilling to accept such radical treatment, particularly if they still have a mobile wrist joint. For this reason, the concept of *radial osteotomy* is an appealing one, since it leaves some degree of wrist mobility.

In theory, a radially based, closing-wedge osteotomy should decompress the radiocarpal joint, at the same time giving significant pain relief as a result of the "osteotomy effect." Furthermore, it seems possible that the radiocarpal ligaments may be tightened by shifting their origin proximally, thus improving the stability of the carpus. To date, this procedure has only been carried out in five patients (Figure 12-15), but the results are encouraging. I believe this procedure may have a place in the management of selected patients with type 3 rotary instability of the scaphoid.

Chapter 12

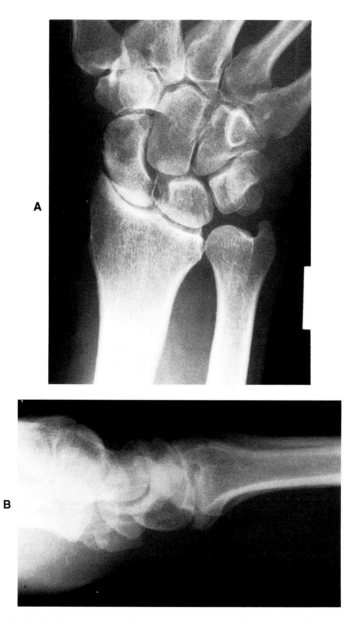

Figure 12-15. Radial osteotomy for symptomatic arthritis secondary to subluxation of the scaphoid (type 3). **A,** Posteroanterior x-ray film shows localised radiocarpal osteoarthritis. **B,** The carpal collapse deformity is best seen on the lateral view.

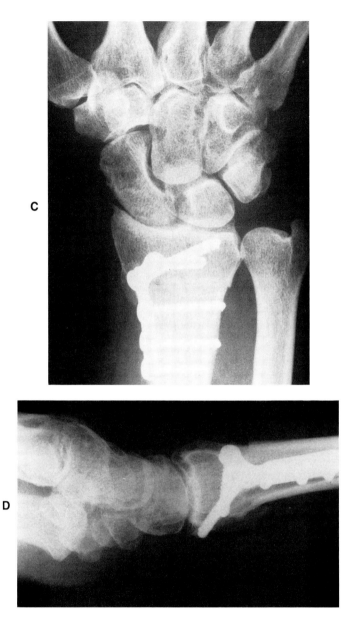

Figure 12-15, cont'd. C and **D,** Films taken 3 months after shortening radial osteotomy show sound bony union with adequate decompression of the radiocarpal joint and apparent improvement in carpal alignment. The patient reports excellent pain relief and maintains his preoperative range of wrist motion.

REFERENCES

1. Herbert TJ, Faithfull RG, McCann DJ, Ireland J. Bilateral arthrography of the wrist. J Hand Surg 15B:233, 1990.
2. Blatt G. Capsulodesis in reconstructive hand surgery: Dorsal capsulodesis for the unstable scaphoid and volar capsulodesis following excision of the distal ulna. Hand Clin 3:81, 1987.
3. Watson HK, Hempton RF. Limited wrist arthrodeses. I. The triscaphoid joint. J Hand Surg 5:320, 1980.
4. Watson HK, Goodman ML, Johnson TR. Limited wrist arthrodeses. II. Intercarpal and radiocarpal combinations. J Hand Surg 6:223, 1981.

The Future

I sincerely hope that the day will come when open reduction and internal fixation are accepted as the treatment of choice for the majority of scaphoid fractures. I believe that this approach will reduce the incidence of major complications and will considerably improve the prognosis for wrist function. Of course, it will be necessary to demonstrate that surgery can produce predictable long-term results, without significant early or late complications.

There is still room for improvement in the techniques for internal fixation of the scaphoid. The operation would be much simpler if we had fine, flexible implants that could be introduced through small skin incisions and yet provide rigid fixation. Reduction of the fracture could be achieved arthroscopically, so that the joint would not need to be opened. It seems likely that future generations of implants will be made from biodegradeable materials, although I am not convinced that these will offer significant advantages over current materials such as titanium, which appears to be highly biocompatible.

Improved diagnostic methods may include the use of routine arthroscopic examination of the wrist in all cases of significant trauma. MRI may assist in diagnosing the early stages of avascular necrosis, before collapse and deformity have occurred, in which case new techniques of bone revascularisation may be used to reverse the disease process.

Reconstruction of the scaphoid will always be necessary as long as acute fractures remain undiagnosed. This problem will be overcome only by educational programs designed to increase awareness that the "sprained wrist," particularly in athletes, actually may be a scaphoid fracture.

The Future

I believe that it would be relatively simple to develop instruments for harvesting bone grafts from the iliac crest by closed methods. I have tried using the Cloward instrumentation for this but have met with little success. Although vascularised bone grafts may be useful in selected cases, I doubt whether their routine use will be justified. Similarly, it will be years before we know whether artificial bone grafts can ever function as well as autogenous bone.

On the question of arthroplasty, there is a real need for improved implants, both for total and for partial replacement of the scaphoid bone. The ideal implant should be stabilised by firm attachment to the adjacent carpal bones. The material should resemble bone, yet the surface properties should be similar to those of hyaline cartilage. Allografts provide the most obvious solution to this problem. Although these have already been used with some success for partial replacement of the scaphoid, the surgical technique is a demanding one, and the long-term results are not yet known.

Limited intercarpal fusions are currently in vogue and the concept behind them is an appealing one. However, the clinical results of this procedure are seldom as good as the x-ray appearance would lead one to expect. Many of my patients continue to complain of persistent pain and loss of wrist function after limited intercarpal fusion. I suspect that the pain arises from increased stress on the unfused joints. If this is so, then these joints are likely to become arthritic, and I suspect many of these patients will eventually need to have their wrists fused.

Total arthroplasty of the wrist is an attractive alternative to fusion but has yet to stand the test of time, particularly in younger patients. It is likely to be some years before a reliable implant becomes available, and I suspect that resurfacing techniques, not bone resection and prosthetic replacement, will provide the best solution.

It is hard to imagine how the operation of wrist fusion could be improved upon except by avoiding it completely! My aims in writing this book will have been achieved the day that wrist fusion is no longer considered as a treatment option for the fractured scaphoid.

Index

A

Accident, motorcycle, 28, 29
Acute compartmental syndrome, 30
Allograft, 131
Anatomical snuff-box, tenderness in, 2, 30
Arch, dorsal radial carpal, 14
Arthritis
 radial styloidectomy and, 140
 rotary subluxation and, 176, 179, 180
 surgery for, 189-191
Arthrodesis of wrist, 151-153
Arthrography
 rotary subluxation and, 182
 ununited fracture and, 38
Arthroplasty, 145-149
Arthroscopy in rotary subluxation, 184
Avascular necrosis, 121-138
 after internal fixation, 88-90
 bone scan for, 38
 complications of, 136-137
 diagnosis of, 124-125
 partial Silastic replacement for, 131-136
 of proximal pole, 16
 staging of, 95
 treatment of, 126-131
Avulsion injury
 avascular necrosis after, 16
 ulnar styloid and, 23

B

Blood supply, 14, 16
Bone graft
 fibrous union and, 98-99
 ischaemia and, 125
 for malunion, 159
 nonunion after, 128-129
 pseudarthrosis and, 105-109
Bone growth stimulator, 129
Bone scan, 38, 39
 avascular necrosis and, 125
Bone screw, Herbert, 78-83
 pseudarthrosis and, 109-110
 rotary subluxation and, 186
Bony versus fibrous union, 47
Bupivacaine, 105

C

Capsule contracture, volar, 31
Capsule repair, 84
Carpal arch, dorsal radial, 14
Carpal collapse deformity
 avascular necrosis and, 122, 125
 dorsiflexion deformity and, 36, 37
 fusion with arthroplasty for, 145-149
 natural history of, 49
 nonunion and, 31
 pseudarthrosis and, 100-101
 rotary subluxation and, 182
Carpal instability, pseudarthrosis and, 44

Index

Carpectomy, proximal row, 150-151
Carpentry, bone, 107-109
Casting, 2-3, 5-6
   internal fixation versus, 59
   nonunion and, 7, 58
   stable fracture and, 52, 53
Child, 163-172
   complications and, 170-171
   diagnosis and, 166
   management of fracture, 166-169
Chronic rotary subluxation of scaphoid, 189
Clamp, jig, 79-81
Classification of fractures, 62-66
Clinical fracture, 56
Closed treatment of fracture, 47
Closing-wedge osteotomy, 189
Closure of wound, 84
Collapse deformity
   carpal
      avascular necrosis and, 122, 125
      dorsiflexion deformity and, 36, 37
      fusion with arthroplasty for, 145-149
      natural history of, 49
      nonunion and, 31
      pseudarthrosis and, 100-101
      rotary subluxation and, 182
   scaphoid, 47, 49
Compartmental syndrome, 30
Complete fracture, 63; see also Unstable fracture
Complex fracture dislocation, 74
Compression fracture of radius, 23
Compression screw fixation, 78-83
Computed tomography, 38
Contracture, volar capsule, 31
Cyst in fibrous union, 96
Cystic changes in avascular necrosis, 125

D

Deformity
   carpal collapse; see Carpal collapse deformity
   dorsiflexed intercalated segment instability, 17, 20
   dorsiflexion, 36, 37
   rotary subluxation and, 176
   scaphoid collapse, 47, 49
Delayed union, 69-90
   complications of, 88-90
   dorsal approach for, 74-76
   dorsolateral approach for, 74
   features of, 65-66
   internal fixation and, 77-84
   postoperative management of, 84-87
   reduction and, 76
   volar approach and, 70-74
Denervation, wrist, 145
DISI; see Dorsiflexed intercalated segment instability
Dislocation
   complex, 74
   rotary subluxation and, 180
   of Silastic prosthesis, 137
   transscaphoid-perilunate fracture, 23
      examination of, 30
Distal oblique fracture, 63
Dorsal approach, 74-76
   proximal pole fracture and, 112
   Silastic replacement and, 135
Dorsal radial carpal arch, 14
Dorsiflexed intercalated segment instability, 17, 20
Dorsiflexion deformity, 36, 37
Dorsolateral approach, 74
Drilling of bone, 82, 83
Dynamic instability in rotary subluxation, 176, 178, 180
   management of, 184
Dynamometer, Jamar, 32

E

Electrode as growth stimulator, 129
Epidemiology, 6-7
Epinephrine in pseudarthrosis, 105
Excision, osteophyte, 143
Extended volar approach, 74
Extension, nonunion and, 31
Extrinsic ligament, 14, 15

F

FCR tendon; *see* Flexor carpi radialis tendon
Femoral neck fracture, 90
Fibrous tissue, avascular necrosis and, 122
Fibrous union
  bony versus, 47
  features of, 66
  proximal pole fracture and, 117
  staging of, 94
  treatment of, 96-99
Fixation, internal, 77-84
  fibrous union and, 99
  ischaemia and, 125
  Kirschner wire as
    arthroplasty with fusion and, 14
    child and, 167
    fracture reduction and, 76
    pseudarthrosis and, 110
    rigid fixation with, 77
    rotary subluxation and, 186
  for malunion, 159
  proximal pole fracture and, 118
  pseudarthrosis and, 101, 109-111
  rotary subluxation and, 186
  wrist fusion and, 152
Flexion at time of impact, 28
Flexor carpi radialis tendon, 70
Fluid, synovial, 46, 47
45-degree oblique view, 34
Fusion
  avoiding of, 49
  intercarpal, 145-149

Fusion—cont'd
  rotary subluxation and, 189
  as salvage procedure, 151-153

G

Graft, bone, 76
  fibrous union and, 98-99
  ischaemia and, 125
  for malunion, 159
  nonunion after, 128-129
  pseudarthrosis and, 105-109
Grip strength, 32
Growth stimulator, bone, 129

H

Haemarthrosis, 30
Healing, avascular necrosis and, 123
Herbert bone screw, 78-83
  pseudarthrosis and, 109-110
  rotary subluxation and, 186

I

Iliac crest bone graft, 99
Imaging, 38-41; *see also* Radiography
Immobilisation, 2-3, 5-6
  child and, 167
  stable fracture and, 52-54
  tubercle fracture and, 57
Impingement, osteophyte, 140
Incomplete fracture; *see* Stable fracture
Instability
  carpal, 44
  intercalated segment
    dorsiflexed, 17, 20
    volar, 38
Intercalated segment instability, 17, 20, 38
Intercarpal fusion, 145-149
Internal fixation, 59-60
  fibrous union and, 99
  ischaemia and, 125

Index

Internal fixation—cont'd
  Kirschner wire as
    arthroplasty with fusion and, 149
    child and, 167
    fracture reduction and, 76
    pseudarthrosis and, 110
    rigid fixation with, 77
    rotary subluxation and, 186
  for malunion, 159
  proximal pole fracture and, 118
  pseudarthrosis and, 101, 109-111
  rotary subluxation and, 186
  technique of, 77-84
  wrist fusion and, 152
Interosseous ligament, short, 14
Interposition of soft tissue, 47
Intramedullary fixation, 78-83
Intrinsic ligament, 14
Irritable wrist, 32
Ischaemic bone, 123, 126, 127

J

Jamar dynamometer, 32
Jig clamps, 79-81
Joint
  midcarpal
    fusion of, 145-149
    ligament rupture and, 174, 183
    shear strain across, 16
    stable versus unstable fracture, 21
    subluxation of, 145-148
  mobility of
    postoperative, 84-85
    rotary subluxation of, 186-187
  soft tissue repair and, 84

K

Kienböck's disease of lunate bone, 125
Kirschner wire
  arthroplasty with fusion and, 149
  child and, 167
  fracture reduction and, 76
  pseudarthrosis and, 110

Kirschner wire—cont'd
  rigid fixation with, 77
  rotary subluxation and, 186

L

Lateral x-ray examination, 36, 37
Ligament
  anatomy of, 14, 15
  midcarpal joint and, 174
  radiocarpal, 84
  radioscaphocapitate, 47
  scapholunate
    arthrography and, 182
    dorsal approach for, 74
    rupture of, 21
    untreated rupture of, 177
  severed, 16-17
Locking in rotary subluxation, 180
Lunate bone, Kienböck's disease of, 125

M

Magnetic resonance imaging, 40, 41
  avascular necrosis and, 125
Malunion, 155-161
  child and, 170
Marcaine, 105
Mechanism of injury, 20-24
Midcarpal joint
  fusion of, with arthroplasty, 145-149
  ligament rupture and, 174
    arthrography of, 183
  shear strain across, 16
  stable versus unstable fracture, 21
  subluxation and, 145-148
Mobility of joint
  postoperative, 84-85
  rotary subluxation and, 186-187
Mobility of wrist, 16-17
Motorcycle accident, 28, 29

N

Natural history of scaphoid fracture, 43-49

Neck, femoral, 90
Necrosis, avascular, 121-138
  after internal fixation, 88-90
  bone scan for, 38
  complications of, 136-137
  diagnosis of, 124-125
  partial Silastic replacement for, 131-136
  of proximal pole, 16
  staging of, 95
  treatment of, 126-131
Nonunion
  after internal fixation, 88
  casting and, 7, 58
  child and, 164-170
  examination for, 31-32
  failed bone grafting and, 128-129
  previous treatment of fracture and, 7
  salvage procedures for, 139-154
    arthroplasty and intercarpal fusion as, 145-149
    osteophyte excision as, 143
    proximal row carpectomy as, 149-150
    radial styloidectomy as, 140-143
    wrist denervation as, 145
    wrist fusion and, 151-153
  synovial fluid and, 46
  treatment of, 91-120
    fibrous, 96-99
    proximal pole fracture and, 112-120
    pseudarthrosis and, 100-112
    stable versus nonstable, 92-95

O

Oblique fracture, 63
Oblique view of wrist, 34
Open reduction of unstable fracture, 59-61
Osteoarthritis
  arthroplasty for, 145-149

Osteoarthritis—cont'd
  radial styloidectomy and, 140
  rotary subluxation and, 176
Osteology, 12-13
Osteophyte
  excision of, 143
  radial styloidectomy and, 140
Osteoporosis, 65
Osteotomy
  avascular necrosis and, 132
  for malunion, 159
  pseudarthrosis and, 103-104
  rotary subluxation and, 189, 191

P

Pain, wrist denervation and, 145
Palmar vessels, 14
Panscaphoid osteoarthritis, 145-149
Partial Silastic replacement, 131-137
Perilunate fracture dislocation, transscaphoid-, 23
  examination of, 30
  features of, 64
Plaster cast, 2-3, 5-6
  internal fixation versus, 59
  nonunion and, 7, 58
  stable fracture and, 52, 53
Preiser's disease, 16, 123
Prosthesis
  arthroplasty with fusion and, 149
  avascular necrosis and, 130-131
Proximal pole
  avascular necrosis of, 16
    bone scan of, 39
    treatment of, 129-131
  fracture of
    child and, 168, 169
    dorsal approach for, 74
    features of, 64
    mechanism of, 21, 22
    tenderness and, 30
    treatment of, 112-120
  pseudarthrosis of, 101

Proximal pole—cont'd
  volar approach to, 73
Proximal row carpectomy, 150-151
Pseudarthrosis, 36, 37
  bone scan of, 39
  characteristics of, 93
  features of, 66
  natural history of, 44
  radial styloidectomy and, 140, 143
  staging of, 94-95
  swelling in, 30
  treatment of, 100-112
    bone graft and, 105-109
    internal fixation for, 109-111
    surgical principles in, 100-102
    technique for, 102-104
  unstable, 35
    natural history of, 47, 49

R

Radial artery, 14
Radial carpal arch, dorsal, 14
Radial deviation view, 33, 34
Radial osteotomy for rotary
    subluxation, 190-191
Radial styloidectomy, 140-143
Radiocarpal ligament repair, 84
Radiography
  avascular necrosis and, 125
  child and, 164-170
  classification of fractures and, 62
  complications of surgery and, 89-90
  diagnosis and, 32-38
  fusion with arthroplasty and,
    146-148
  history of injury and, 2-3, 4
  ischaemia and, 127
  Kirschner wire and, 110
  limitations of, 24
  malunion and, 156-158
  nonunion and, 8-9, 128-129
  postoperative, 86, 87
  proximal pole fracture and, 113-119

Radiography—cont'd
  pseudarthrosis and, 144
  rotary subluxation and, 180, 182,
    183
    preoperative, 186
    screw loosening in, 187
  scapholunate ligament rupture, 177
  Silastic replacement and, 135
  stable fracture and, 52, 53, 54,
    55
  wrist fusion and, 152
Radiolunate ligament, 14
Radioscaphocapitate ligament
  trapping of, 47
  volar, 14
Radius, compression fracture of, 23
Range of motion, 31
Reduction of fracture, 76
Resting splint, 85
Reversible ischaemia of scaphoid, 123,
    127
Rotary subluxation, 173-192
  diagnosis of, 180-184
  surgery for, 184-191
Rupture, ligament
  midcarpal joint and, 174
  scapholunate, 21
    arthrography in, 182
    untreated, 177

S

Salvage procedures for nonunion,
    139-154
  arthroplasty and intercarpal fusion
    as, 145-149
  osteophyte excision as, 143
  proximal row carpectomy as,
    149-150
  radial styloidectomy as, 140-143
  wrist denervation as, 145
  wrist fusion and, 151-153
Scan, bone, 38, 39
  avascular necrosis and, 125

Scapholunate ligament
  dorsal approach for, 74
  rupture of
    arthrography in, 182
    mechanism of injury in, 21
    untreated, 177
Scintigraphy of scapholunate
    ligament rupture, 182
Screw, Herbert bone, 78-83
  pseudarthrosis and, 109-110
  rotary subluxation and, 186
Shear strain
  across midcarpal joint, 16
  transscaphoid-perilunate fracture
    and, 23
Short interosseous ligament, 14
Silastic prosthesis, 131-137
Silicone synovitis, 137
Skeletally immature patient,
    163-172
  complications in, 170-171
  diagnosis in, 166
  management of, 166-169
SLAC procedure for rotary
    subluxation, 189
Soft tissue
  blood supply and, 16
  repair of, 84
  tubercle fracture and, 57
  union and, 47
  volar approach and, 73
Splint
  postoperative, 85
  stable fracture and, 53
  tubercle fracture and, 57
Sprain of wrist, 2
  child and, 164
Stabilisation, 101
Stable fracture
  classification of, 62
  natural history of, 46
  treatment of, 52-55
Stable scaphoid nonunion, 92-93

Staging of nonunion, 94-95
Staple fixation, 77-78
Static instability in rotary
    subluxation, 176, 178
Stimulator, bone growth, 129
Strain, shear, 16
Strength, grip, 32
STT fusion contraindicated, 189
Styloidectomy, radial, 140-143
Subcapital fracture of femoral neck,
    90
Subluxation, rotary, 173-192
  diagnosis of, 180-184
  surgery for, 184-191
Surgery for scaphoid fracture, 69-90
  complications of, 88-90
  dorsal approach of, 74-76
  dorsolateral approach of, 74
  internal fixation in, 77-84
  postoperative management of,
    84-87
  reduction and, 76
  volar approach of, 70-74
Swanson prosthesis
  arthroplasty with fusion and,
    149
  avascular necrosis and, 131
Swelling, 30
Synovitis
  Silastic prosthesis and, 137
  swelling and, 30
Synovium in nonunion, 46, 47

T

Tenderness, 2, 30
Tendon in wrist fusion, 152-153
Tortional force, 28
Transscaphoid-perilunate fracture
    dislocation, 23
  examination of, 30
  features of, 64
Trapping of radioscaphocapitate
    ligament, 47

Index

Tubercle
  child and, 164
  fracture of
    clinical, 56, 57
    features of, 62
    mechanism of, 21, 22
  tenderness and, 30

U

Ulnar deviation view, 33, 34
Ulnar side of wrist, tenderness on, 30
Union
  fibrous
    bony versus, 47
    features of, 66
    proximal pole fracture and, 117
    staging of, 94
    treatment of, 96-99
  malunion, 155-161
    in child, 170
  nonunion; see Nonunion
Unstable fracture, 17, 20
  classification of, 63-66
  natural history of, 46
  treatment of, 57-61
Unstable pseudarthrosis, 35
  natural history of, 47, 49
Unstable scaphoid nonunion, 92-93
Unstable wrist, rotary subluxation and, 180
Ununited fracture; see Nonunion

V

Vascular supply, 14, 16
Vascularised graft, 125

VISI; see Volar intercalated segment instability
Volar approach to surgery, 70-74
  pseudarthrosis and, 103-104
  Silastic replacement and, 131-134
Volar capsule contracture, 31
Volar extrinsic ligament, 15
Volar intercalated segment instability, 38
  after internal fixation, 89
Volar radiocarpal ligament repair, 84
Volar radioscaphocapitate ligament, 14
Volar resting splint, 85

W

Waist fracture
  child and, 164
  complete, 63
  incomplete, 62
  mechanism of, 21
Wire, Kirschner
  arthroplasty with fusion and, 149
  child and, 167
  fracture reduction and, 76
  internal fixation and, 77
  pseudarthrosis and, 110
  rotary subluxation and, 186
Wound closure, 84
Wrist capsule repair, 84
Wrist denervation, 145
Wrist fusion, 151-153